# Bone Grafting Techniques for Maxillary Implants

# Bone Grafting Techniques for Maxillary Implants

Karl-Erik Kahnberg

Professor and Head of Department of Oral and Maxillofacial Surgery
Gothenburg University
Sweden

*with contributions from*
Lars Rasmusson
Associate Professor
Department of Oral and Maxillofacial Surgery
Gothenburg University
Sweden

Göran Zellin
Consultant
Clinic of Odontology
Gothenburg
Sweden

Blackwell
Munksgaard

Published on behalf of Astra Tech
by Blackwell Munksgaard

Published by
Blackwell Munksgaard, a Blackwell Publishing company
Editorial Offices:
Blackwell Publishing Ltd, 9600 Garsington Road, Oxford OX4 2DQ, UK
Tel: +44 (0)1865 776868
Blackwell Publishing Professional, 2121 State Avenue, Ames, Iowa 50014-8300, USA
Tel: +1 515 292 0140
Blackwell Publishing Asia, 550 Swanston Street, Carlton, Victoria 3053, Australia
Tel: +61 (0)3 8359 1011



First published 2005 by Blackwell Munksgaard

Library of Congress Cataloging-in-Publication Data
Kahnberg, Karl-Erik.
Bone grafting techniques for maxillary implants / Karl-Erik Kahnberg.
p. ; cm.
Includes bibliographical references and index.
ISBN 1-4051-2994-8 (alk. paper)
1. Maxilla – Surgery. 2. Implants, Artificial. 3. Bone-grafting.
[DNLM: 1. Dental Implantation, Endosseous – methods. 2. Maxilla – surgery. WU 640 K12b 2005] I. Title.

RD526.K24 2005
617.5′220592 – dc22
2004019236

ISBN 1-4051-2994-8

A catalogue record for this title is available from the British Library

Set in 10/13pt Palatino
by SNP Best-set Typesetter Ltd., Hong Kong
Printed and bound in Denmark
by Narayana Press, Odder

The publisher's policy is to use permanent paper from mills that operate a sustainable forestry policy, and which has been manufactured from pulp processed using acid-free and elementary chlorine-free practices. Furthermore, the publisher ensures that the text paper and cover board used have met acceptable environmental accreditation standards.

For further information on Blackwell Munksgaard, visit our website:
www.dentistry.blackwellmunksgaard.com

# Contents

*List of Figures* vii

*Biography* xiii

*Introduction* xv

**1 Biological Principles of Bones** **1**
1.1 History 1
1.2 Indications and terminology 1
1.3 Bone sources 1
1.4 Healing principles and success factors 2
1.5 Future possibilities 3

**2 Implant Integration in Normal Bone and Bone Grafts** **5**
2.1 Introduction 5
2.2 Measurements of implant stability 6
2.3 Implant integration in autogenous bone grafts 7

**3 Grafting Procedures** **11**
3.1 Bone graft from the iliac crest 11
3.2 Bone graft from the tibia 13
3.3 Chin grafts 14
3.4 Mandibular angle graft 15
3.5 Graft from the maxillary tuberosity 17
3.6 Bone collecting devices 18

**4 Onlay Bone Grafting** **19**
4.1 Minor bone graft with particulated bone 19
4.2 Minor bone graft in block form 21
4.3 Major onlay bone grafts in block form 23
4.4 To be mentioned 29

**5 Inlay Bone Grafting** **31**
5.1 Nasal inlay grafting 31
5.2 Maxillary sinus grafting (sinus lifting) 33
5.3 Impaction of alveolar bone into the maxillary sinus 47
5.4 Maxillary osteotomy with interpositional bone graft 47

**6 Segmental Osteotomy for Bone Augmentation Procedures** **57**
6.1 Indication 57
6.2 Surgical technique 59

**7 Distraction Osteogenesis for Augmentation of the Alveolar Process** **63**
7.1 Indication 63
7.2 Surgical technique 66

**8 Complications** **69**
8.1 Grafting sites 69
8.2 Onlay grafting 69
8.3 Inlay grafts 70

**9 Bone Substitutes in Maxillary Reconstruction Procedures** **73**
9.1 Bone substitutes 73

**10 Summary and Conclusion** **75**

*References* 79

*Further Reading* 84

*Index* 89

# List of Figures


| | |
|---|---|
| **Figure 2.1** | A transducer connected to an implant fixture. To be able to compare different implants, the unit Implant Stability Quotient (ISQ) has been developed. ISQ corresponds to 50 Hz, 6 |
| **Figure 2.2** | Stability evaluation for implants integrated in grafted and ungrafted bone, 9 |
| **Figure 2.3** | Removal torque values for the same implants, 9 |
| **Figure 3.1** | Grafting procedures, 11 |
| **Figure 3.2** | Soft tissue dissection down to the iliac crest, 12 |
| **Figure 3.3** | The top of the iliac crest is elevated to gain access to the medial surface, 12 |
| **Figure 3.4** | The medial aspect of the iliac bone is exposed, 12 |
| **Figure 3.5** | The size of the bone graft is prepared, 12 |
| **Figure 3.6** | The medial bone block graft is mobilized and removed, 12 |
| **Figure 3.7** | The block graft obtained, 13 |
| **Figure 3.8** | Incision closed with continuous intracutaneous suture, 13 |
| **Figure 3.9** | Tibia graft, 13 |
| **Figure 3.10** | Bone graft from the tibia, 13 |
| **Figure 3.11** | The grafting site after removal of block graft and spongious bone, 14 |
| **Figure 3.12** | Intraoral grafting procedures, 14 |
| **Figure 3.13** | Surgical exposure of the chin between the mental foramina. A block graft is obtained, 15 |
| **Figure 3.14** | Another design of block graft from the chin region, 15 |
| **Figure 3.15** | Surgical exposure of the chin and graft donor sites after harvesting bone with a trephine drill, 15 |
| **Figure 3.16** | Bone graft from the mandibular angle via a sagittal split approach in soft and hard tissue, 16 |
| **Figure 3.17** | The bone block is split out buccally, 16 |
| **Figure 3.18** | The inferior alveolar nerve is medial to the bone graft region, 16 |
| **Figure 3.19** | Bone graft material from the mandibular angle and trephine material from the chin, 16 |
| **Figure 3.20** | Bone mill for particulation of the bone graft, 17 |
| **Figure 3.21** | Details of particulated bone graft, 17 |
| **Figure 3.22** | BoneTrap™ for collection of particulated bone graft when preparing the fixture site, 18 |
| **Figure 4.1** | Onlay bone grafting, 19 |
| **Figure 4.2** | Extraction site with only the palatal cortex left, 20 |
| **Figure 4.3** | Implant with most of the threads exposed buccally, 20 |

**Figure 4.4** Particulated bone and bone graft from the BoneTrap™ collected during preparation of the implant site and covering the implant, 20
**Figure 4.5** Bone graft healing after five months. A layer of mature bone is covering the implant, 20
**Figure 4.6** Fixture exposure after anchorage in the marginal area and the nasal bone, 20
**Figure 4.7** Exposed threads covered with bone graft from BoneTrap™, 21
**Figure 4.8** Thin bone lamellae now covering the fixture after four to five months healing, 21
**Figure 4.9** Minor bone graft block, 21
**Figure 4.10** Bone deficiency in a case of aplasia, 22
**Figure 4.11** A small circular bone graft is taken from the chin, 22
**Figure 4.12** The graft is modeled and secured with a plate screw, 22
**Figure 4.13** Bone material from BoneTrap™ is packed around the onlay graft, 22
**Figure 4.14** Bone healing after five months. The graft is integrated with only minor resorption, 22
**Figure 4.15** Implant installed in the grafted bone, 22
**Figure 4.16** Onlay bone grafting, 23
**Figure 4.17** Patient with severely resorbed maxilla, 24
**Figure 4.18** Vestibular incision prior to onlay block grafting of the whole maxilla, 24
**Figure 4.19** The bony maxilla is exposed and the nasal mucosa lifted carefully, 24
**Figure 4.20** Horseshoe shaped graft is obtained from the iliac bone below the iliac crest, 25
**Figure 4.21** The bone graft is modeled to fit onto the alveolar crest in all directions, 25
**Figure 4.22** Light compression of the soft tissue by the acrylic stent connected to the zygoma, 25
**Figure 4.23** Acrylic wafer with posterior extension to avoid trauma to the grafted region, 25
**Figure 4.24** The onlay bone graft is connected to the alveolar crest by simultaneous insertion of the implant screws, 25
**Figure 4.25** Careful attention is taken to remove all sharp edges of the graft, 25
**Figure 4.26** The incision is closed with continuous suturing, 26
**Figure 4.27** Soft tissue healing after ten days, 26
**Figure 4.28** Implants in place in the upper jaw, 26
**Figure 4.29** Radiograph of bone graft and implants, 26
**Figure 4.30** Bone graft and implants after healing for six months, 27
**Figure 4.31** Prosthetic reconstruction after one year, 27
**Figure 4.32** Graft with osteosutures, 27
**Figure 4.33** A defect in the alveolar process in the right posterior maxilla after trauma, 27
**Figure 4.34** The clinical situation, 28
**Figure 4.35** Onlay block graft from the hip connected to the residual bone by means of the implants, 28

**Figure 4.36** Postoperative radiograph showing demineralized bone graft. The implants seem to be without support, 28

**Figure 4.37** One year later the bone graft contour is clearly visible, 28

**Figure 4.38** Split crest technique for the alveolar process, 29

**Figure 5.1** Inlay bone grafting, 31

**Figure 5.2** Nasal inlays, 32

**Figure 5.3** The nasal mucosa in the nasal aperture is carefully lifted, 32

**Figure 5.4** Bone graft is pressed into the nasal cavity below the nasal mucosa, 32

**Figure 5.5** The bony height of the alveolar process increased by 5–6 mm, 32

**Figure 5.6** The nasal inlays combined with onlay grafts on the thin alveolar crest, 32

**Figure 5.7** Local sinus lift procedure, 34

**Figure 5.8** Intraoral radiograph showing the available bone height after extraction of tooth 16, 35

**Figure 5.9** Surgical exposure of the alveolar crest, 35

**Figure 5.10** Infracture of a bony window with simultaneous lifting of the sinus membrane and insertion of the implant, 35

**Figure 5.11** Radiograph showing the implant in position, 36

**Figure 5.12** One year postoperative. Radiograph showing remodelling of graft material, 36

**Figure 5.13** Radiograph of extraction site after removal of second premolar, 36

**Figure 5.14** Elevation of mucoperiosteal flap and removal of bone close to the sinus membrane, 36

**Figure 5.15** Clinical view of implant touching and lifting the sinus membrane, 36

**Figure 5.16** Bone material from BoneTrap™ is packed around the exposed part of the implant, 36

**Figure 5.17** Radiograph of implant in place where half of the implant is placed into the sinus cavity, 37

**Figure 5.18** Exposure for abutment connection four months later shows satisfactory bone healing, 37

**Figure 5.19** One-stage grafting, 38

**Figure 5.20** Clinical view of posterior maxilla with elevation of mucoperiosteal flap and osteotomy performed according to the window technique using a round bur, 38

**Figure 5.21** Elevation of the sinus membrane and infracture of the bony window, 38

**Figure 5.22** The sinus recess is created for the bone graft by lifting the bone window and sinus mucosa, 38

**Figure 5.23** Bone graft from iliac crest (cortical and cancellous) is positioned in the sinus recess and implants inserted, 38

**Figure 5.24** Clinical view of bone graft and implants in relation to the sinus membrane and window, 38

**Figure 5.25** Suturing of the flap. Note that incision line is positioned palatally of the crest, 39

**Figure 5.26** Bone healing six months later, 39

**Figure 5.27** Two-stage procedure, 40

**Figure 5.28** Patient with loss of teeth in the left posterior maxilla, 40
**Figure 5.29** Panoramic X-ray shows inadequate bone volume beneath sinus on the left side, 40
**Figure 5.30** Sinus lifting with bone graft from the iliac crest. The graft is immobilized with osteosutures. The bone window is used as an onlay graft, 40
**Figure 5.31** Uncomplicated healing of the soft tissues, 40
**Figure 5.32** Radiograph showing the bone graft in position, 41
**Figure 5.33** Tomograph showing the amount of bone augmentation, 41
**Figure 5.34** Clinical view after four months healing, 41
**Figure 5.35** Surgical guide for positioning of implants in the grafted bone, 41
**Figure 5.36** Tomography of implants in place in the bone graft, 42
**Figure 5.37** Radiograph of the implants in the available graft material, 42
**Figure 5.38** Clinical view of definitive superstructure, 42
**Figure 5.39** Bone window infractured for sinus lifting procedure in the right posterior maxilla, 43
**Figure 5.40** A space is created inferior to the bone window with the sinus membrane on top of window, 43
**Figure 5.41** Particulated bone graft is placed below the bony window, 43
**Figure 5.42** Implants inserted after four months of healing, 43
**Figure 5.43** Bridge connected to implants, 43
**Figure 5.44** Radiograph of right posterior maxilla showing sinus cavity occupying the alveolar process, 44
**Figure 5.45** Tomography showing the residual bone volume, 44
**Figure 5.46** Tomography after bone graft placement and wires, 44
**Figure 5.47** Panoramic view showing the bone graft reconstruction of the right posterior maxilla, 44
**Figure 5.48** Bony union of graft material after four months, 45
**Figure 5.49** Preparation of implant site and guide pins, 45
**Figure 5.50** Radiograph showing position of implants, 45
**Figure 5.51** Implants placed in grafted bone, 45
**Figure 5.52** Bridge construction on four implants, 45
**Figure 5.53** Clinical view of bone window in right posterior maxilla, 46
**Figure 5.54** Infracture of bone window with elevation of sinus membrane, 46
**Figure 5.55** Bone graft from the right mandibular angle (cortical) positioned below the bone window and sinus mucosa. Osteosuture is introduced around the graft material, 46
**Figure 5.56** Space below the cortical graft is filled with particulated bone, 46
**Figure 5.57** Osteosutures are tightened to keep the bone graft in place, 46
**Figure 5.58** Impaction of alveolar bone with the osteotome technique, 47
**Figure 5.59** Maxillary osteotomy, 48
**Figure 5.60** Extreme atrophy of the maxilla, 49
**Figure 5.61** Vestibular incision marked, 49
**Figure 5.62** Mucoperiosteal flap elevated and the bony nasal aperture exposed. Note the nasal floor at the level of the crest, 49

**Figure 5.63** Down-fracture of the resorbed thin maxilla. Sinus cavities and the nasal floor are exposed, 49

**Figure 5.64** Bone graft from iliac crest is positioned in sinus cavities and nasal floor and is secured with osteosutures, 49

**Figure 5.65** The maxilla is anteriorly and inferiorly repositioned and immobilized with two plates; one on each side of the nasal aperture, 49

**Figure 5.66** Continuous sutures for closure of vestibular incision, 50

**Figure 5.67** Healing of soft tissues after two weeks, 50

**Figure 5.68** Lateral radiograph preoperatively, 50

**Figure 5.69** Lateral radiograph after bone grafting and anterior repositioning, 50

**Figure 5.70** Bone graft and osteosutures in the down-fractured maxilla, 50

**Figure 5.71** The grafted maxilla is secured with plates on both side of the nasal cavity, 50

**Figure 5.72** Panoramic radiograph showing an extremely resorbed upper jaw, 51

**Figure 5.73** Lateral view further illustrates the lack of bone in the maxilla and the retrognathic position, 51

**Figure 5.74** Lateral radiograph after maxillary osteotomy Le Fort I with interpositional bone graft and anterior repositioning of the maxilla, 51

**Figure 5.75** Clinical picture of bone graft healing after 4–5 months, 51

**Figure 5.76** Panoramic radiograph after grafting procedure, 52

**Figure 5.77** Implants inserted in the grafted maxilla, 52

**Figure 5.78** Lateral radiograph of the anteriorly repositioned maxilla with implants, 52

**Figure 5.79** Panoramic view with implants in place, 52

**Figure 5.80** Panoramic radiograph of patient with advanced periodontal and cariogenic disease in his residual dentition of the upper jaw. Note the traumatic loss of the anterior teeth, 53

**Figure 5.81** Lateral radiograph showing a retrognathic position of the upper jaw partly due to the traumatic injury, 53

**Figure 5.82** The situation after maxillary osteotomy with anterior repositioning of the maxilla and interpositional bone graft, 53

**Figure 5.83** Rehabilitation with implants and bridge, 54

**Figure 5.84** Panoramic radiograph after implant rehabilitation, 54

**Figure 5.85** Clinical situation after prosthetic rehabilitation, 54

**Figure 5.86** The case illustrates an almost total absence of bone in the maxilla. Lateral radiograph shows very retropositioned maxilla, 55

**Figure 5.87a** Scanora tomography showing absence of bone beneath the sinus cavity, 55

**Figure 5.87b** The same projection with bone graft in place, 55

**Figure 5.88** Panoramic view after bone grafting, 56

**Figure 5.89** Lateral radiograph after bone grafting showing a better sagittal relation, 56

**Figure 5.90** The patient after prosthetic rehabilitation, 56

**Figure 5.91** Clinical view of bridge reconstruction, 56

**Figure 6.1** Segmental osteotomy, 57

**Figure 6.2** Traumatic injury with loss of teeth and alveolar bone in the maxillary anterior region, 57
**Figure 6.3** Panoramic view of the situation, 58
**Figure 6.4** Vestibular incision with exposure of the alveolar process and segmental osteotomy of the edentulous portion, 58
**Figure 6.5** Bone graft from the chin is positioned in the gap after elevation of the segment to increase the alveolar height, 58
**Figure 6.6** Lateral radiograph visualizing the bone graft site, 58
**Figure 6.7** Implants inserted in elevated segment, 59
**Figure 6.8** Bone material from BoneTrap™ smoothing the bone surface, 59
**Figure 6.9** Panoramic radiograph of implants in place, 59
**Figure 6.10** A patient with fibrous dysplasia where the posterior edentulous maxilla had increased in height preventing occlusal rehabilitation, 60
**Figure 6.11** The clinical situation with no space between dentition in the lower jaw and the opposing alveolar crest, 60
**Figure 6.12** Surgical intrusion of segment and insertion of implants, 61
**Figure 6.13** Segmental osteotomy with bone graft, 61
**Figure 7.1** Distraction, 63
**Figure 7.2** Clinical situation in a patient after traumatic loss of teeth and bone, 63
**Figure 7.3** Vestibular incision and exposure of the alveolar process, 63
**Figure 7.4** Segmental osteotomy performed with a thin oscillating saw blade, 64
**Figure 7.5** Thin plates (stop plate and distraction plate) are secured in the bone segment and the alveolar base. The distraction screw is introduced through the segment, 64
**Figure 7.6** Clinical view after healing period, 64
**Figure 7.7** After distraction for one week the segment is elevated, 64
**Figure 7.8** The final situation with distracted segment, 64
**Figure 7.9** Insertion of implants, 64
**Figure 7.10** Radiograph showing implants in place, 65
**Figure 7.11** Rehabilitation with a bridge, 65
**Figure 7.12** Tomography before the start of distraction, 65
**Figure 7.13** Tomography showing 7–8 mm distraction osteogenesis, 66
**Figure 7.14** Distraction technique, 67
**Figure 8.1** Partial exposure of large onlay graft. Secondary healing with loss of some of the graft material, 70
**Figure 8.2** Trauma from denture with exposure of cover screws and part of the implants, 70
**Figure 8.3** Wound dehiscences after crestal incision in connection with sinus grafting, 71
**Figure 8.4** Sinusitis with fistula after sinus lifting procedure, 71
**Figure 8.5** Sequestration of bone graft in maxillary sinus, 71
**Figure 9.1** Patient with bone deficiency around inserted implant, 73
**Figure 9.2** Bio-Oss® granules are used to improve stability and increase width of alveolar crest, 73

# Biography

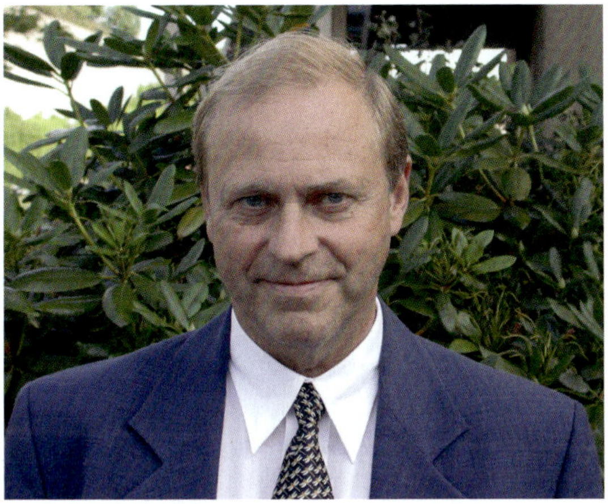

Professor Karl-Erik Kahnberg is Head of the Department of Oral and Maxillofacial Surgery, at the Sahlgrenska Academy, Gothenburg University, Sweden. He is also the clinical director for the maxillofacial unit at the Public Dental Health University Clinics in Gothenburg.

He has a major clinical interest in maxillofacial surgery, especially orthognathic surgery, where his surgical experience has been useful in solving demanding implant reconstruction cases. The use of bone grafts from varying sites has been extremely valuable to treat bone deficient areas with implant reconstructions. He has wide experience in all kinds of implant surgery which has also been documented in a number of scientific publications.

Numerous international courses, focusing on bone grafting procedures in connection with implant treatment, have been attended by dentists and specialists from all over the world. Professor Kahnberg has frequently been invited to lecture at these international conferences and postgraduate education programs. His far-reaching clinical experience of bone grafts in implant reconstruction is now collected in this book for the interested surgeon to share his surgical knowledge.

# Introduction

Implant rehabilitation using titanium screw-shaped implants has been an extremely important innovation as reported in numerous publications over the years. In the beginning of the implant era, the anterior mandible was the primary implant site because it demonstrated remarkably good results in long-term follow-up studies (Adell *et al.* 1981; Albrektsson *et al.* 1986; Arvidsson *et al.* 1998; Makkonen *et al.* 1997). Long-term results point to the impressive stability and safety of the procedure. Over time, the use of implants in other sites such as the maxilla and posterior mandible have shown almost the same predictability (Adell *et al.* 1990a; Lekholm *et al.* 1994). New designs of implants are continuously introduced into the market, often with little or no scientific documentation; however, the screw-shaped implant has the longest and most reliable documentation available today.

The mandible demonstrates the highest predictability of results, especially in the frontal region between the mental foramina. It is possible to consider immediate loading of the implants due to the mandible's initial stability compared to the maxilla, which in most cases is considerably more problematic in relation to bone quality and quantity. Patients with poorer bone quality and less quantity of bone have been excluded from implant treatment for a long time. However, the advent of bone reconstruction of deficient areas, both in the mandible and the maxilla, has improved the possibility of treatment for the bone deficient patient. Different bone grafting techniques have been developed and orthognathic surgical procedures adapted to the special demands of implant surgery have meant that most bone problems can now be solved.

One-stage techniques employ grafting and implant surgery in the same operative procedure, whereas two-stage techniques employ grafting and reconstruction in one procedure and implant surgery in a second phase. Depending on the amount of bone graft necessary, the source for the graft can been chosen from different parts of the body. If only small amounts of bone graft are necessary for the implant site, bone may be harvested from the mandible or maxilla, for example, from the mandibular symphysis region, mandibular angle and ramus, maxillary tuberosita or adjacent to the implant site. Using bone collectors, it is also possible to filter out bone powder during drilling of the implant site. Bone substitutes or demineralized bone in combination with autogenous bone material have also been shown to function well in alveolar bone reconstruction (Henry *et al*. 1996; Pinholt *et al*. 1992).

Bone grafts have been used in oral and maxillofacial surgery for a long time in for the reconstruction of the jaw bones to rectify facial deformities, for pre-prosthetic reconstruction, and also for reconstruction after trauma and tumour damage. Where the bone graft has been used as a bridge over bony defects or filling out defects, the results have been good, but when used as an augmentation material for pre-prosthetic reconstruction, more progressive resorption of the graft has occurred. Onlay bone grafting in connection with implant surgery was the first method developed to overcome the bone deficient maxilla, however, the graft in an onlay position with or without a denture on top of it has not been a predictable procedure (Gordh 1998). The graft was most frequently taken from the iliac crest, initially as a horseshoe-shaped graft in one or two pieces. The graft was modeled to fit the alveolar crest and stabilized with the implants into the residual bone.

This book will be of interest both to experienced surgeons and residents in oral and maxillofacial surgery. Surgical techniques for the rehabilitation of severe bone deficiencies in the maxilla are described and detailed illustrations of patient cases are provided.

# 1 Biological Principles of Bone

## 1.1 History

Repairing and restoring bone defects has a long history. The surgeons of the pre-Incan period used gold and silver plates and shells as grafting materials to repair trephine holes in the skull 3000 years BC. Trephination – the removal of a circular section of bone from the skull – is the oldest known surgical intervention. Dr Philip von Walter is credited in 1821 as being the first surgeon to use bone autografts for reconstruction of the remaining defect after a trephination in the skull. The term 'autograft' implies transplantation of bone tissue from one site to another, within the same individual. Bone transplantation has been a common surgical procedure since the early 1920s.

## 1.2 Indications and terminology

The general indications for using a bone graft are when there is a need to: (i) replace missing bone; and/or (ii) enhance bone formation, in order to restore form and function. Many types of materials have been used and tested to replace missing bone during the last century, for example, banked bone (allograft; bone from individuals within the same species), xenografts (bone derived from other species), ceramics such as hydroxyapatite, metals, corals and plastics. Today, however, fresh autogenous cancellous and cortical bone remain the most widely used materials and are still considered the 'gold standard' in bone grafting and other bone regenerative procedures. Autografts have superior osteogenic capacity compared to both allografts and xenografts, and since they are derived from the patient's own tissue, the risk of rejection is minimized.

## 1.3 Bone sources

The most frequently used site for bone harvest is the iliac crest. In general, this site can supply enough volume of both cortical and cancellous bone for different reconstructive purposes in the maxillofacial region. Other sites also used, although less commonly, are the tibia, fibula and the ribs. When only a small amount of bone is needed, it can be harvested from the chin or at the anterior aspect of the mandibular ramus. The last two sites can, however, only contribute compact bone.

A bone graft may be of two types: free vascularized (i.e. a graft with vessels to be connected with vessels at the recipient bed), or free non-vascularized. The vascularized bone graft may have higher chances of survival but, on the other hand, this type of grafting is more time-consuming and more expensive.

## 1.4 Healing principles and success factors

The success of a bone grafting procedure is dependent on many factors. The first of these is the inherent biological activity of the graft, i.e. the number of living cells and their cellular products, including proteins stored within the matrix. The second factor is the capability of the graft to elicit an osteogenic response in the tissues at the recipient bed, and a third consideration should be the ability of the graft to support and promote in-growth of new bone derived from the surrounding tissues at the recipient bed of the host. A non-vascularized graft is also completely dependent on the surrounding tissue at the recipient bed for its revascularization.

Another important factor, also contributing to the success of grafting, is the mechanical properties at the recipient site. Actions at the interface between the graft and the host tissues may jeopardize the subsequent revascularization of the graft. Taken together, the success of grafting is dependent on a sequence of cellular, biochemical and biomechanical events that follow a rather predictable schedule. Graft incorporation will not occur if there is a problem with any of these events or with the order in which they occur.

The sequence of events that take place during the process of bone graft incorporation mimics the process seen during fracture healing. Both fractures and the transplantation of a bone graft result in injuries to the local vessels with bleeding and the formation of a hematoma. This hematoma activates a clotting cascade and, subsequently, fibrin clot formation. Within the next seven days, an inflammatory response will develop with invasion of different neutrophilic cells, lymphocytes and plasma cells, i.e. an acute inflammatory process. Some in-growth of new vessels may also be observed.

At the end of the first week after the grafting procedure, a parallel process will begin. The clot will organize and turn into fibrous granulation tissue which unites the grafted bone with the recipient bone. The granulation tissue also attracts phagocytozing inflammatory cells such as macrophages and multinuclear giant cells, as well as osteoclasts to remove dead bone and debris. At the end of the second week angiogenesis commences.

During the first couple of weeks after a bone grafting procedure, there are only small differences in the response towards cortical and cancellous grafts. The principal difference involves revascularization. Cancellous grafts may, at least partly, be revascularized within a few hours after the transplantation, mainly due to anastomoses between injured host vessels and graft vessels, but also because revascularization occurs through open marrow spaces, of which there are many in cancellous bone. Complete revascularization of a cancellous graft may be completed within two weeks. In contrast, revascularization of cortical grafts is much slower. By two weeks, the cortical graft is pierced with channels, produced by the osteoclasts to allow new vascular ingrowth, a process that will subside at six weeks.

Transplanted cortical bone has approximately 50% less physical strength than the host bone at the recipient site due to the channels produced by the osteoclasts. The grafted bone will continue to be weaker, at least during the first year after the transplantation, after which time it will become as strong as the bone at the recipient bed. Grafted cortical bone particles may not entirely be replaced with host bone at the recipient bed, but grafted cancellous bone will be completely replaced by new host bone within the first year after transplantation.

## 1.5 Future possibilities

During the last decade, extensive improvements have been made in tissue engineering and tissue regeneration, especially within the skeletal field (see Zellin 1998, for review). Gene technology has allowed us to sequence many growth factors and other proteins involved in both formation and turn over of bone; these have been produced by recombinant techniques. One group of proteins, bone morphogenetic proteins (BMPs), have shown themselves to be able to regenerate both skeletal tissue and to induce new bone formation in both animals and humans. One crucial factor with this type of treatment is the route of administration. BMPs and other growth factors of possible interest are proteins, and hence need a carrier to remain as inactive proteins for some time after administration into the tissue. The carrier must be designed to release the proteins at intervals and to then be degraded relatively fast and with the least possible tissue reaction. A solution to this carrier problem has not yet been found, but when it does become available, this new technique has the potential to reduce the need for bone grafting procedures, thereby reducing cost as well as the risk of donor site morbidity and patient discomfort.

# 2 Implant Integration in Normal Bone and Bone Grafts

## 2.1 Introduction

When an implant site is prepared, the surgical trauma will cause a preprogrammed healing response that aims at complete repair of the wound by new bone formation, remodeling and maturation. As a result of implant installation, a hematoma is formed which initiates a clotting reaction. Residual bone debris produced during drilling and implant installation is deposited around the implant site. The debris will subsequently be surrounded by macrophages and multinuclear giant cells and/or be covered by new bone. After some weeks, woven bone is formed both near the implant and some distance away in the medullary cavity. A study with mice has found that the woven bone will gradually remodel into a mature lamellar bone in 3–4 weeks (Nanci *et al.* 1994), but in humans this maturation takes several months.

The early bone tissue response to unloaded, screw-shaped titanium implants inserted in the rabbit tibia was studied by Sennerby and colleagues (1993). The animals were sacrificed according to a pre-determined schedule so that histologic sections were available after 3 days, 7 days, 14 days, 28 days, 42 days, 90 days and 180 days. A cellular response was evident 3 days after implantation when mesenchymal cells were seen migrating into the injury area. Multinuclear giant cells were commonly observed on the implant surface after 7 days. Woven bone formation occurred at a distance from the surface at the endosteal bone surfaces and in the collagen matrix in the marrow compartment. With time, the amount of bone increased and approached the implant surface to fill the threads of the implant screw, in parallel with a decreasing number of multinuclear giant cells. Remodeling of the interface seemed to be complete by 90 days.

Most studies on the ultrastructure of the bone-titanium interface show that there is an unmineralized or partly mineralized zone separating the titanium surface from the bone (Albrektsson *et al.* 1982, 1985; Linder *et al.* 1989; Sennerby *et al.* 1992; Nanci *et al.* 1994). The dimension of this zone varied between the different studies but was generally less than 500 nm. Thus, the ultrastructural studies on the bone-titanium interface and other biocompatible metals indicate that the stability of such implants is due to mechanical strength rather than to a true bond between the bone and metal.

A number of studies have addressed the bone response to titanium implants with modified surfaces and designs. Some of these studies have indicated increased bone-implant contact with increased surface roughness (Buser *et al.* 1991; Goldberg *et al.* 1995; Gotfredsen *et al.* 1995). Wennerberg (1996) and Rasmusson *et al.* (2001) showed that a certain degree of surface roughness may result in more bone-implant contacts, while surfaces that are too smooth or too rough may lead to inferior integration.

Histology of clinically retrieved implants has revealed a high amount of bone-titanium contact and bone fill in the threads 1–16 years after loading (Albrektsson *et al.* 1993). The interface of these implants consisted of a mixture of bone (about 85%) and bone-derived soft tissue, which probably reflected normal bone morphology.

The incorporation of a bone graft and the integration of implants are both complex healing situations, which must result in direct contact between the remodelled bone graft and the implant. In contrast to normal bone, the preparation of an implant site in a free bone graft will probably not initiate a repair process, due to the interrupted microcirculation and rapid cell death. To evaluate and understand implant integration in this complex healing situation, different parameters such as stability measurements and histology are crucial.

## 2.2 Measurements of implant stability

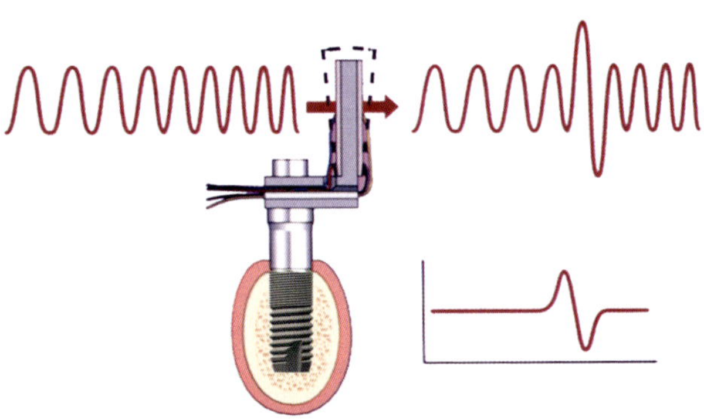

**Figure 2.1** A transducer connected to an implant fixture. To be able to compare different implants, the unit Implant Stability Quotient (ISQ) has been developed. ISQ corresponds to 50 Hz.

One of the most frequently used parameters for evaluation of osseointegration is histology. Histomorphometry – the measurement of the degree of bone-implant contact and amount of bone filling the implant screw's threads – is a way to describe implant stability. However, it is difficult to obtain this type of evaluation from patients, and hence is seldom used. A successful technique for implant stability measurements has been developed by Meredith and colleagues (1996a). A small transducer is attached to the implant and the resonance frequency measured. The resonance frequency is determined by the stiffness of the transducer-implant-bone complex and the distance from the transducer to the first bone-implant contact. Using resonance frequency analysis (RFA) increased implant stability with time has been demonstrated, probably due to an increased stiffness of the bone-implant interface, which in turn is a result of bone formation, remodelling and maturation.

Another technique used for evaluation of osseointegration is the removal torque test. This technique measures the strength of the interface in shear, while the RFA method is more of a bending test. The methods are partly but not fully related to each other. For instance, O'Sullivan *et al.* (2000) compared the stability of threaded implants with different surface roughness using both removal torque tests and RFA. Twelve weeks after grafting, they found no differences in primary or secondary stability with RFA but statistically more removal torque was required to unscrew the rough implants when compared to the machined ones. This difference may be explained by the fact that RFA measures the marginal bone support which should be similar for test and control sites, while removal torque is determined by the degree of interlock, which is highly influenced by the properties of the implant surface. In clinical studies, the only repetitive, non-invasive technique for stability measurements is RFA.

## 2.3 Implant integration in autogenous bone grafts

Experimental studies have shown that titanium implants will integrate both in particulated bone grafts and block grafts. In rabbits, Albrektsson (1980a, b) used a specially constructed titanium implant for *in vivo* visualization of the healing of bone grafts. Repeated inspections during the follow-up period revealed that in-growth of new vessels in cancellous and cortical bone took varying amounts of time. In cancellous bone the maximum rate was 0.4–1.2 mm a day, while in cortical bone the maximum rate was 30–40 μm a day. Therefore, a higher degree of resorption can be anticipated for cortical bone than for cancellous bone. However, when using cortico-cancellous bone grafts with the cortical layer facing the periosteum, it can be expected that the cortex will resist a collapse of the graft with ingrowth of soft tissue, thereby retaining original volume and acting as a template for osteogenesis.

Smith and Abrahamson (1974) used bicortical iliac onlay grafts and onlay calvarial bone grafts in rabbits and reported that the bicortical iliac graft had viable surface bone, but the cancellous bone was resorbed after three months. The cortical surfaces were noted to be thinner and the grafts smaller. The calvarial graft, on the other hand, had increased in thickness during the same period. This difference was even more pronounced after one year. One theory for this difference is that bone from the rib, tibial and ilium retain their calcified matrix better when subjected to functional forces like strain or stress. When used as a graft, such bone can be expected to lose more of its calcified matrix compared to the calvarial bone graft, which does not rely on functional loading.

Neukam *et al.* (1989) and Lew *et al.* (1994) have experimentally observed direct contact between onlay iliac bone grafts and Brånemark implants when using simultaneous placement of implants. Neukam *et al.* (1989) used miniature pigs where the premolars were extracted in the mandible. After three months of healing, defects were created in the alveolar crest and free grafts were transplanted from the iliac crest to the defects and fixed with implants. Direct bone-to-implant contact was observed in both the recipient and grafted areas. Lew *et al.* (1994) also used simultaneous placement of bone grafts and implants and in dogs compared the integration of the implants in cortico-cancellous block grafts with integration in cortico-cancellous particulated grafts. The authors found a higher degree of bone density with a higher degree of bone-to-implant contact for the block grafts compared with the particulated grafts, and they concluded that osseointegration of titanium implants developed more rapidly in block grafts compared to particulated grafts.

In an experimental investigation, Shirota *et al.* (1991) studied the effect of simultaneous and delayed placement of HA-coated implants in free bone grafts and observed a higher degree of bone-to-implant contact for the delayed implants. Rasmusson *et al.* (1998) showed that titanium implants, placed simultaneously with an onlay bone graft in the rabbit tibia, integrated with the graft. This gave them greater stability, as measured with resonance frequency analysis and removal torque, compared to ungrafted controls.

In another study, using the same rabbit model and technique (RFA), it was possible to compare simultaneous vs delayed placement of implants in onlay bone grafts. When the bone graft was left to heal before implant placement, the stability of the implant was greater than that achieved with implants placed simultaneously with the bone graft.

There are only a few clinical reports that investigate the histology of implants and autogenous bone grafts. Nyström *et al.* (1993b) presented the histology of one patient who died four months after simultaneous placement of an onlay bone graft and six titanium implants in the maxilla. The bone graft, harvested from the iliac crest, showed signs of resorption, but there were also areas of newly formed bone. There was only a patchy contact between the grafted bone and the implants, with the major part of the interface consisting of soft tissue. However, all implants were clinically stable, as verified at postmortem. In a case report by Piatelli *et al.* (1997) mature bone was observed at the interface of an implant placed eight months after a bone grafting procedure to reconstruct a mandible with discontinuity and removed after 10 months of loading.

Jensen and Sennerby (1998) investigated the histological changes caused by titanium microimplants simultaneously placed in the augmented maxillary sinus using either autogenous grafts or allogenic material. It was evident that implants placed in autogenous bone had a higher degree of bone-to-implant contact after 6 to 12 months of healing, compared to those implanted in allogenic bone. These authors also concluded that simultaneous placement resulted in a low degree of bone-implant contact irrespective of healing time and graft type. A staged protocol seems to be preferable when using autogenous block bone grafts and dental implants.

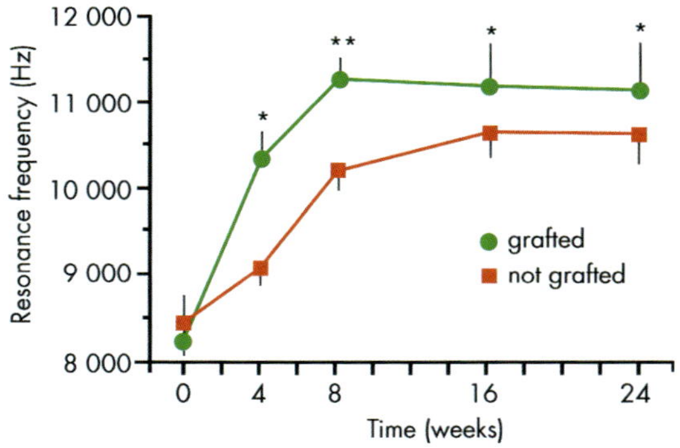


**Figure 2.2** Stability evaluation for implants integrated in grafted and ungrafted bone.

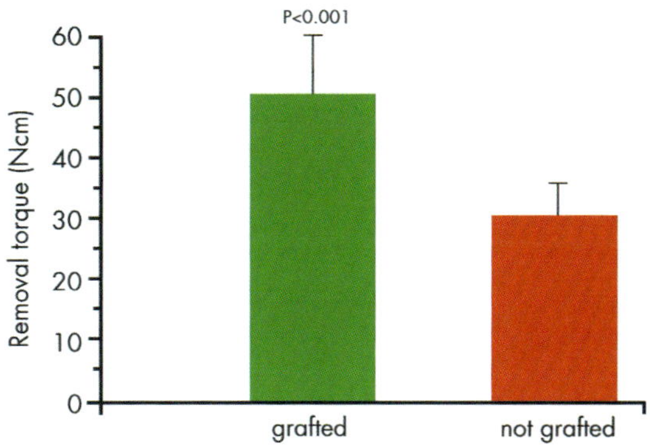


**Figure 2.3** Removal torque values for the same implants.

# 3 Grafting Procedures

## 3.1 Bone graft from the iliac crest

### *3.1.1 Indication*

This procedure is indicated when a large amount of graft material is needed. Cortical as well as cancellous bone may be collected in sufficient amounts to restore severely resorbed maxillae or, for example, when bilateral sinus lift procedures are required and can also be combined with nasal inlays. It is possible to harvest both block grafts and particulated bone of the desired volume and shape.

### *3.1.2 Technique*

The incision line is located just lateral to the bony crest, and extends between 5–15 cm depending on the amount of bone needed. Blunt dissection is used through subcutaneous muscle and adipose tissue down to the periosteum covering the iliac crest. Limiting cuts are made through the periosteum into the bone and a superficial part of the bone crest is elevated. The bony lid is displaced medially and the bone surface exposed on the medial aspect. The desired volume of bone is then harvested in the region between and within the initial stop cuts, although care must be taken not to perforate the full thickness of the iliac bone unless a very significant bone graft is needed. After harvesting, the bone lid is repositioned to restore the initial anatomical

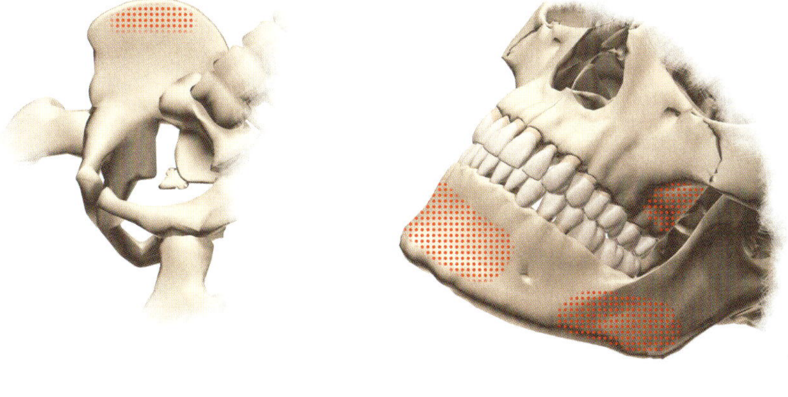

**Figure 3.1** Grafting procedures.

shape of the iliac crest. The graft can of course also be obtained from the lateral surface of the ilium and some surgeons also include the iliac crest in the graft. However, from experience, postoperative problems are very much related to the technique used for the grafting procedure. The less traumatic approach, where anatomical structures are restored as far as possible, will certainly decrease postoperative morbidity.

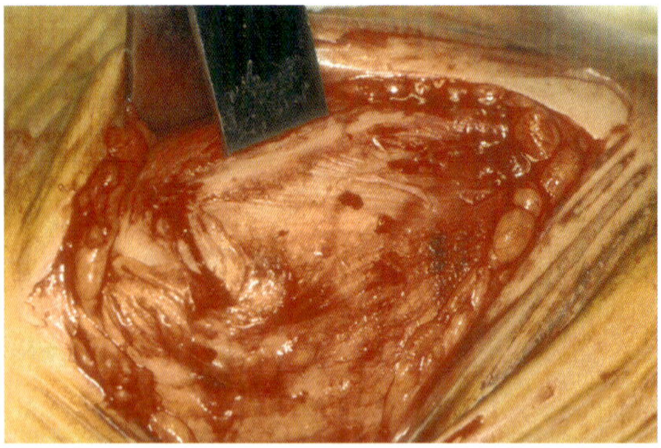

**Figure 3.2** Soft tissue dissection down to the iliac crest.

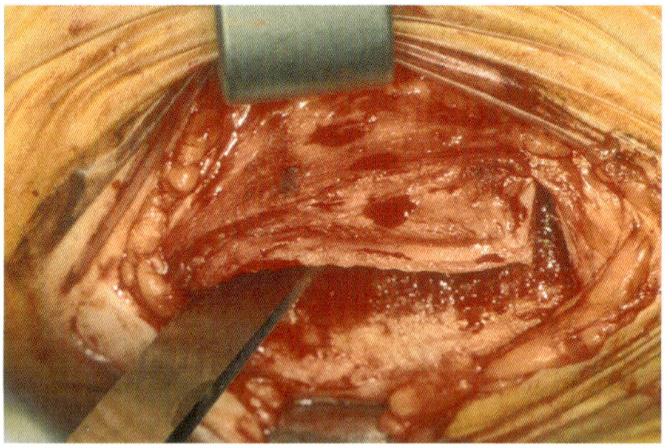

**Figure 3.3** The top of the iliac crest is elevated to gain access to the medial surface.

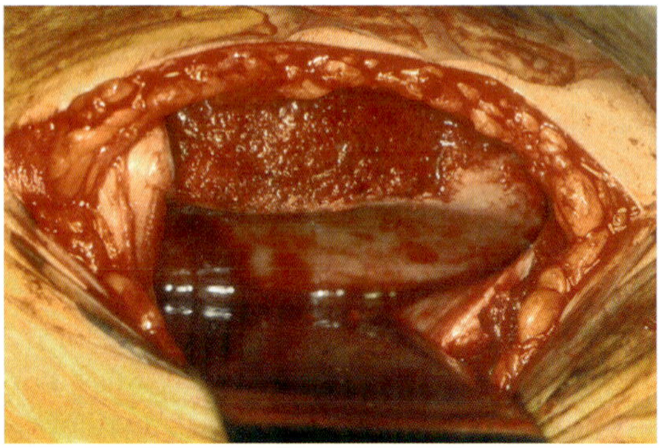

**Figure 3.4** The medial aspect of the iliac bone is exposed.

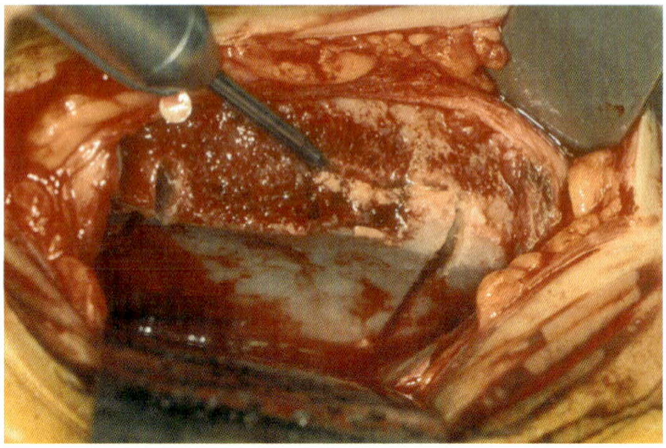

**Figure 3.5** The size of the bone graft is prepared.

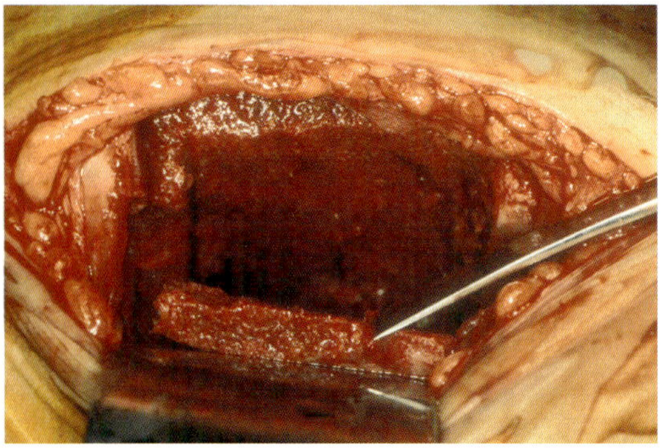

**Figure 3.6** The medial bone block graft is mobilized and removed.

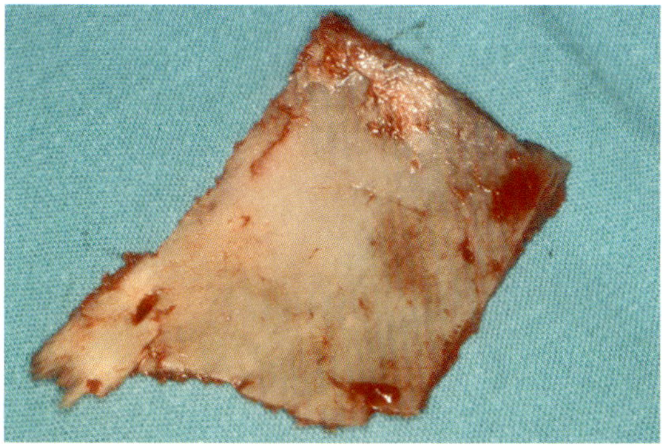

**Figure 3.7** The block graft obtained.

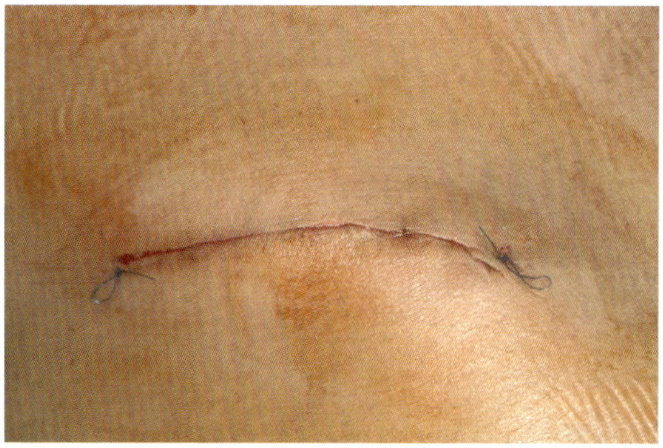

**Figure 3.8** Incision closed with continuous intracutaneous suture.

## 3.2 Tibial grafts

### 3.2.1 *Indication*

Due to the anatomy of the tibia and the cancellous nature of the bone, a limited volume of graft material is available for grafting. This graft is indicated for use in unilateral sinus lift procedures or as onlay grafting material.

### 3.2.2 *Technique*

A semicircular skin incision is made on the anterior aspect of the tibia. A skin and periosteal flap is raised to expose the bony surface. Using a round bur or a Lindemann bur and chisels, a rectangular part of the cortical bone is removed after which access can be gained to the cancellous bone in the marrow space. The cancellous bone is of very good quality with a low lipid content. The periosteum and skin flap is carefully resutured. The patient will experience some pain and should be instructed not to bear weight on the donor leg too much during the first week. Otherwise, the post-operative problems appear to be minor.

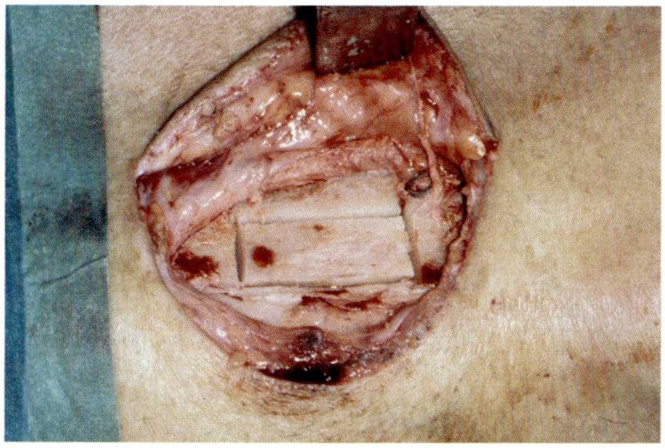

**Figure 3.9** Tibia graft.

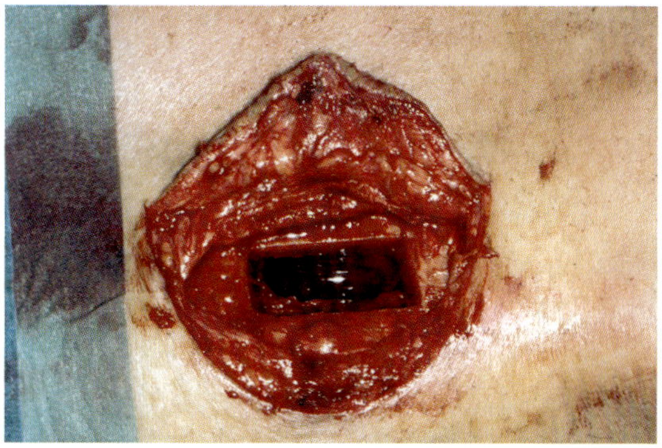

**Figure 3.10** Bone graft from the tibia.

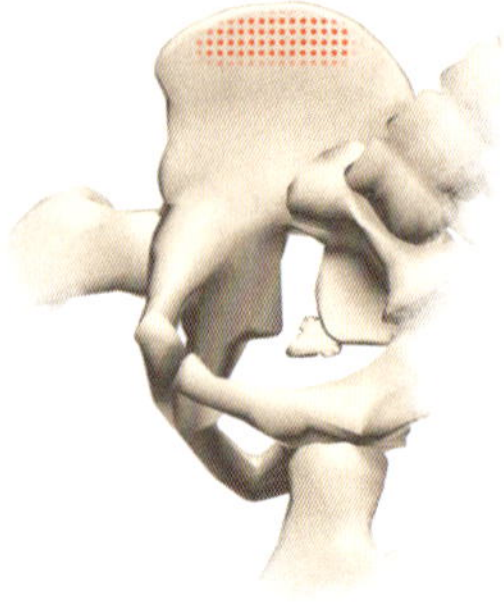

**Figure 3.11** The grafting site after removal of block graft and spongious bone.

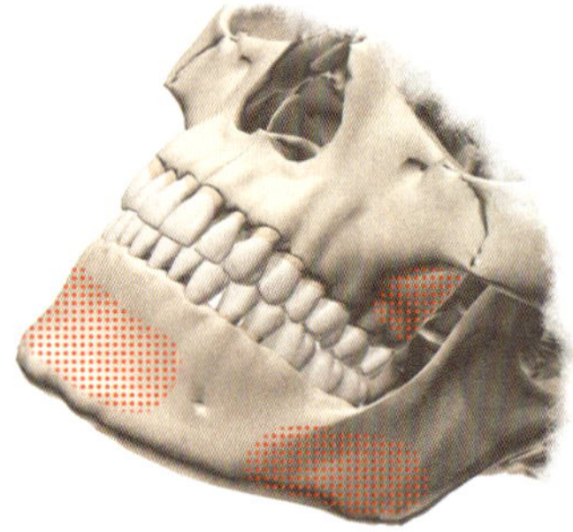

**Figure 3.12** Intraoral grafting procedures.

## 3.3 Chin grafts

### 3.3.1 *Indication*

Due to the limited amount of bone available, this graft is mostly indicated for use in unilateral sinus lifting procedures or onlay grafting for widening of a thin crest.

### 3.3.2 *Technique*

The parasymphyseal region of the chin is used for harvesting chin bone. A vestibular mucosal incision is made with due attention to the fact that the mental nerve may be crossing the area. Blunt dissection is carried out through the mental muscle down to the periosteum, which is sharply cut horizontally. The soft tissue is reflected to expose the bone surface. The bone surface can be exposed from the mental foramen on one side to that on the contralateral side. With a round bur or a Lindemann bur a rectangular bone area is delineated down to the narrow space.

It is of the utmost importance that the area does not approach too closely to the apices of the anterior teeth. A distance of at least 5–10 mm is recommended to assure the vitality of the teeth and also to avoid contact with the anterior branch of the inferior alveolar nerve which could result in traumatic neuralgic pain or even numbness. The inferior border of the bony cut should be at least 2 mm above the inferior border of the mandible.

It is possible to harvest only a very limited volume of cancellous bone from this region. The cortical bone is very hard but can be particulated if necessary. The contour of the graft is suitable for positioning in the sinus recess or used for buccal onlay grafting. The soft tissue is closed in layers with resorbable sutures in the periosteum and muscles and a continuous suture in the mucosa. Patients often have some pain and a degree of discomfort for some time after this procedure.

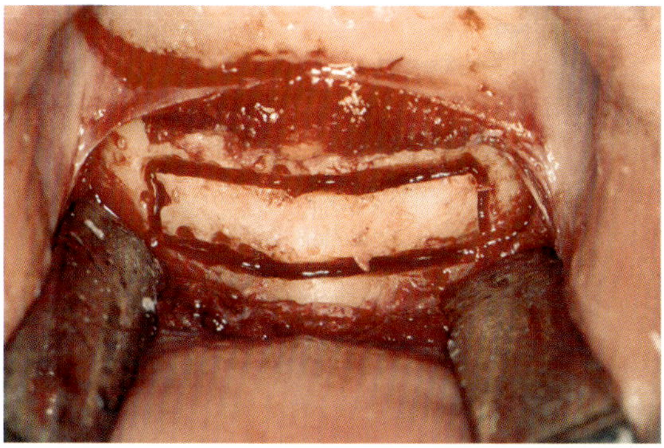

**Figure 3.13** Surgical exposure of the chin between the mental foramina. A block graft is obtained.

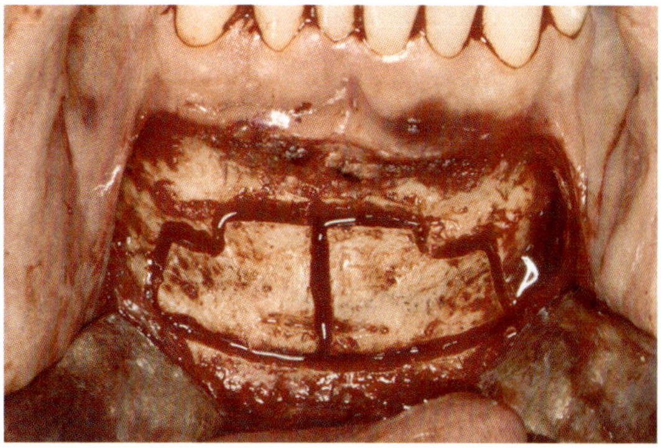

**Figure 3.14** Another design of block graft from the chin region.

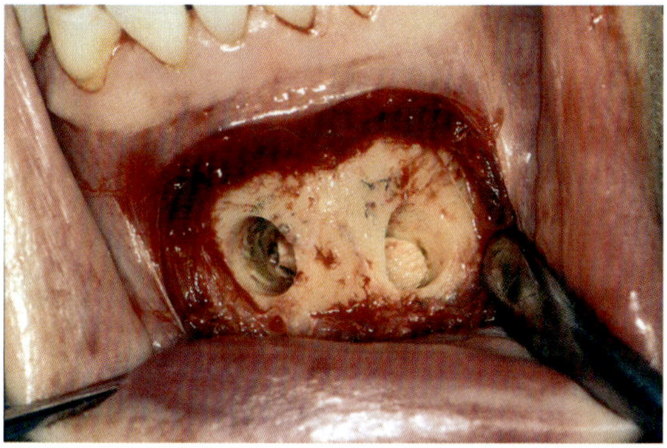

**Figure 3.15** Surgical exposure of the chin and graft donor sites after harvesting bone with a trephine drill.

## 3.4 Mandibular angle graft

### 3.4.1 *Indication*

This graft can be utilized for unilateral and sometimes bilateral sinus grafting procedures, as well as onlay grafting. It is useful in block as well as in particulated form. There are certain limitations to the size of the graft although more material is available than from the chin. Almost no cancellous bone can be harvested from this area.

### 3.4.2 *Technique*

The mucoperiosteal incision is placed lateral to the dental arch leaving 2 mm gingival cuff attached to the distal tooth for suturing. The incision is the same as for a sagittal split operation. The lateral bone surface is exposed by careful reflection of the flap. The extent of the bone graft is assessed and stop cuts made vertically with a Lindemann bur. A horizontal cut then joins the stop cuts, with due caution to prevent the bur from penetrating the central marrow space. Another stop cut is made as far inferior as possible, ensuring that it does not approach the inferior alveolar nerve. The cut should extend a couple of centimetres down, towards the inferior border. The bone block may be split away very carefully with a straight chisel to avoid interference with the alveolar nerve. It should be noted that sometimes the inferior alveolar nerve canal is situated in the cortical bone and has to be released from the graft before harvesting.

After removal of the graft, the soft tissue is closed with continuous sutures. Patients generally experience very little discomfort from this procedure but always demonstrate marked swelling.

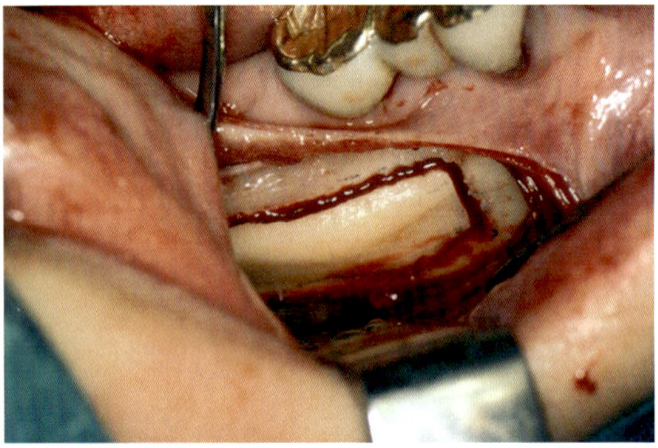

**Figure 3.16** Bone graft from the mandibular angle via a sagittal split approach in soft and hard tissue.

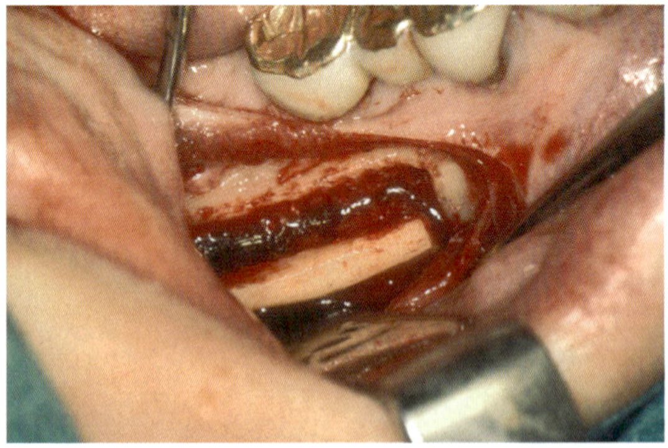

**Figure 3.17** The bone block is split out buccally.

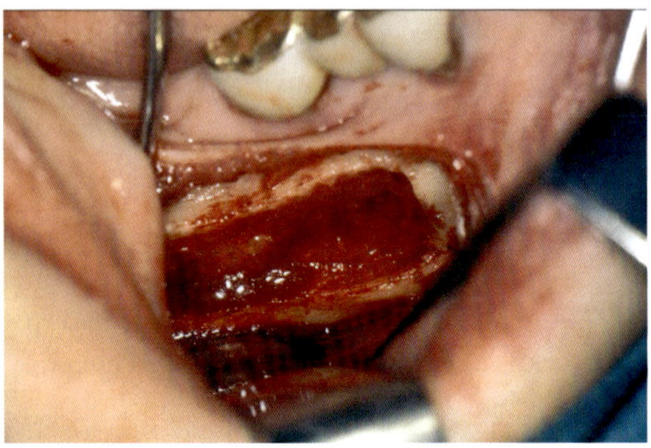

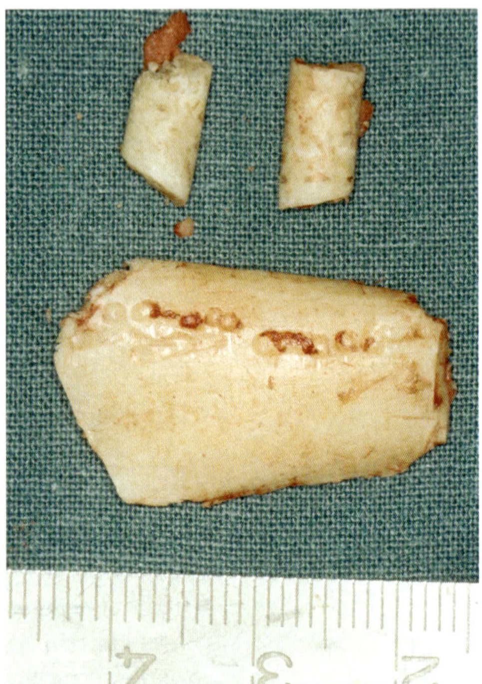

**Figure 3.18** (*above*) The inferior alveolar nerve is medial to the bone graft region.
**Figure 3.19** (*right*) Bone graft material from the mandibular angle and trephine material from the chin.

## 3.5 Graft from the maxillary tuberosity

### 3.5.1 *Indication*

This procedure is only for very limited grafting procedures with no need for cortical bone. Sometimes it can be enough for unilateral sinus lifts, but is typically used for filling minor defects and covering exposed implant threads.

### 3.5.2 *Technique*

A crestal incision is made over the region of the bony tuberosity and a releasing incision located buccally to the molar region. The soft tissue is reflected on both buccal and palatal sides, thus exposing the bony tuberosity. The tuberosity tissue, which has often undergone fatty degeneration, can be harvested with a bone cutter, taking care to avoid getting too close to the adjacent teeth. The soft tissue is contoured and closed with interrupted sutures. The patient experiences little or no discomfort from this procedure.

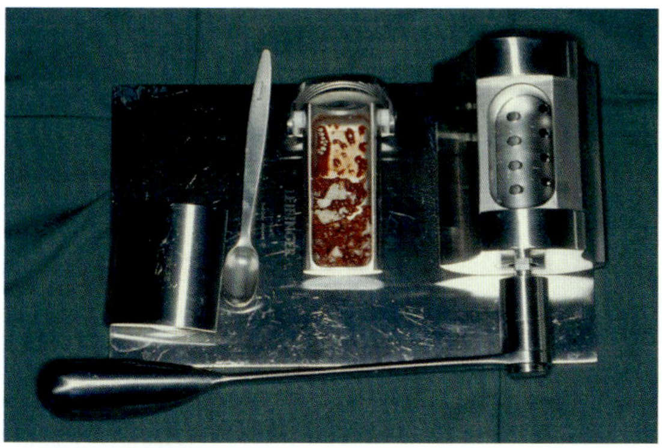

**Figure 3.20** Bone mill for particulation of the bone graft.

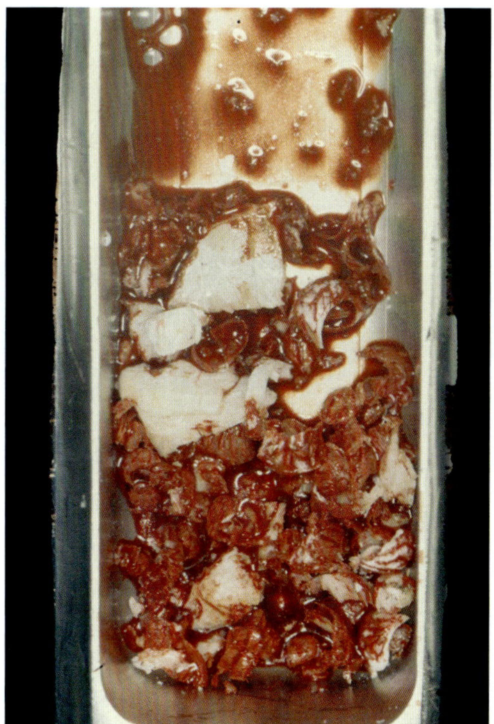

**Figure 3.21** Details of particulated bone graft.

## 3.6 Bone collecting devices

The bone grafting procedures necessary to harvest adequate bone for major reconstructive surgery often require additional surgical training and admittance for general anaesthesia and hospital care. For minor procedures that demand very limited amounts of bone graft, bone collecting devices may be useful. These collect particles of bone during drilling of the implant site. BoneTrap™ (see Figure 3.22) is a disposable filter chamber that can be used for collecting small amounts of bone. Other types of collecting devices such as the 'Safe Scraper' collect the bone by removing the surface layers of the bone adjacent to the implant site. Bone substitutes such as Bio-Oss® or similar materials derived from artificial bone matter or hydroxyapatite material, are used more and more frequently. There are different opinions about their benefit for bone growth but they may serve as a matrix for implant support and are potentially very good as augmentation material in different regions of the mouth.

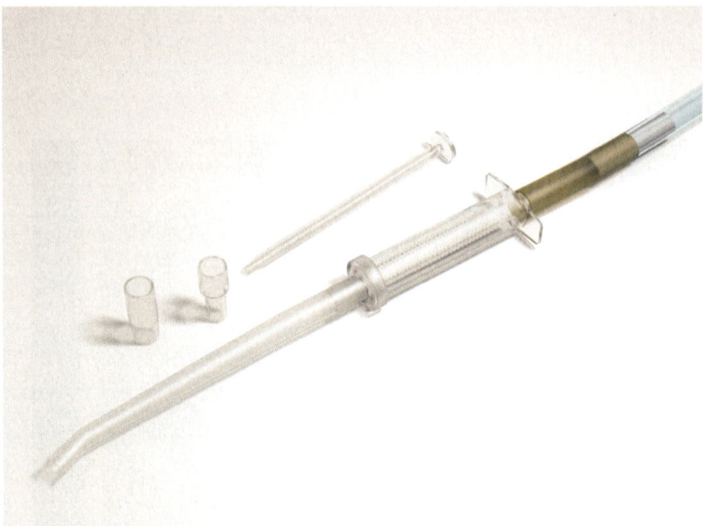

**Figure 3.22** BoneTrap™ for collection of particulated bone graft when preparing the fixture site.

# 4 Onlay Bone Grafting

## 4.1 Minor bone graft with particulated bone

Onlay grafting is a method of increasing bone volume but can also be used to level deformities in the bone contour or to cover dehiscences such as those following traumatic extraction of teeth. In cases where only small amounts of bone material are needed it may be enough to collect bone with a BoneTrap™ during preparation of the fixture site or to take small pieces of bone from an adjacent area such as the tuberosity or nasal spine. In these cases the bone graft does not have a stabilizing effect on the implant but serves instead as a means for improving the esthetic appearance.

The bone particles are placed over the defect with or without a covering membrane. However, it is advisable to use the intact periosteum as an autologous membrane with a suturing technique to keep the bone material in place. It is also recommended to close the flap over the implant and graft material in order not to jeopardize graft healing. Healing before abutment connection is dependent upon the initial stability of the fixture and may take three to six months.

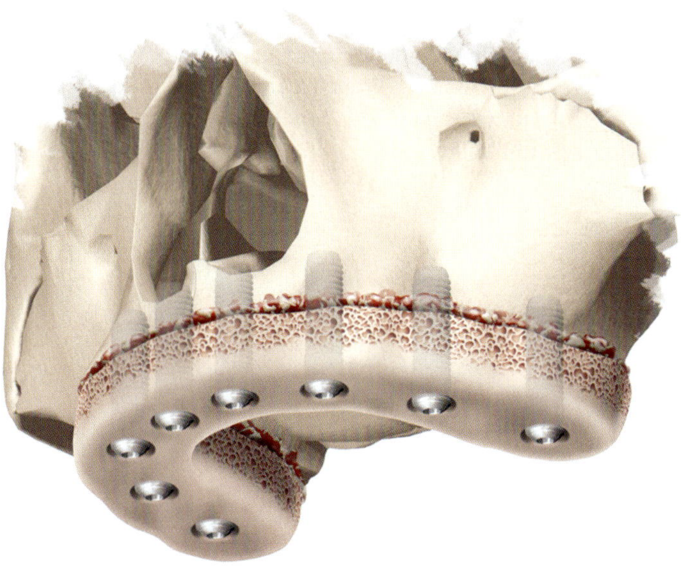

**Figure 4.1** Onlay bone grafting.

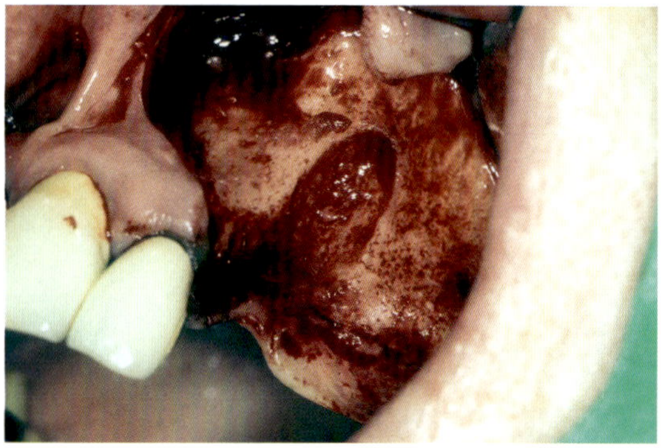

**Figure 4.2** Extraction site with only the palatal cortex left.

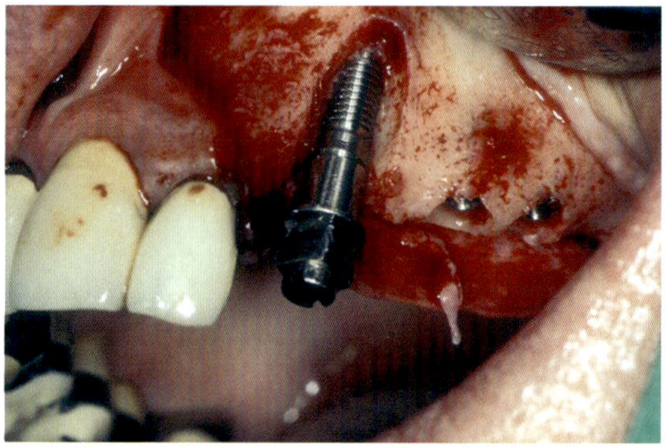

**Figure 4.3** Implant with most of the threads exposed buccally.

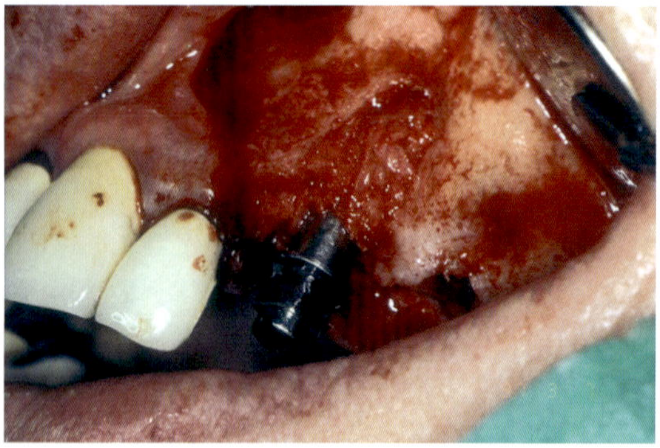

**Figure 4.4** Particulated bone and bone graft from the BoneTrap™ collected during preparation of the implant site and covering the implant.

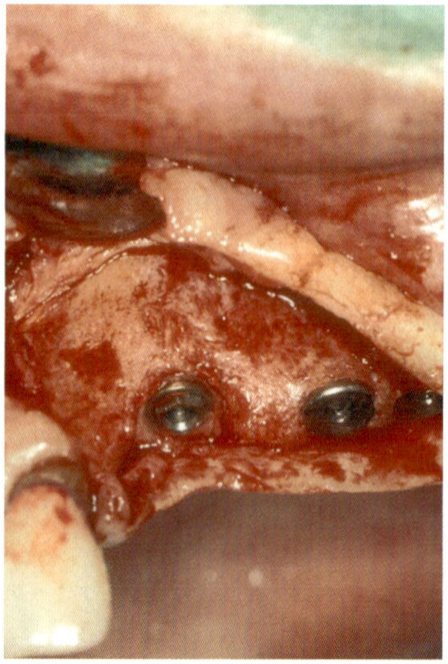

**Figure 4.5** Bone graft healing after five months. A layer of mature bone is covering the implant.

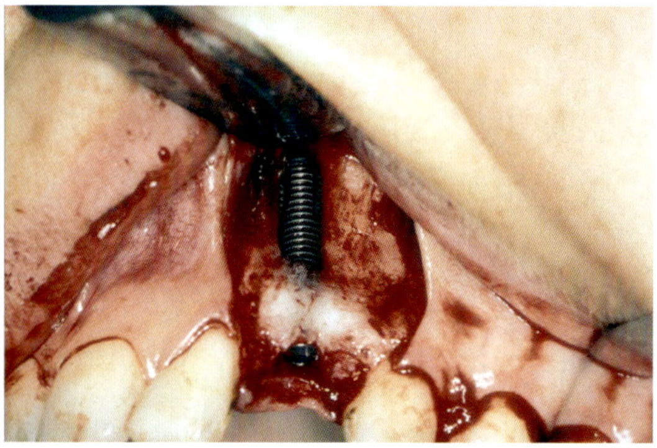

**Figure 4.6** Fixture exposure after anchorage in the marginal area and the nasal bone.

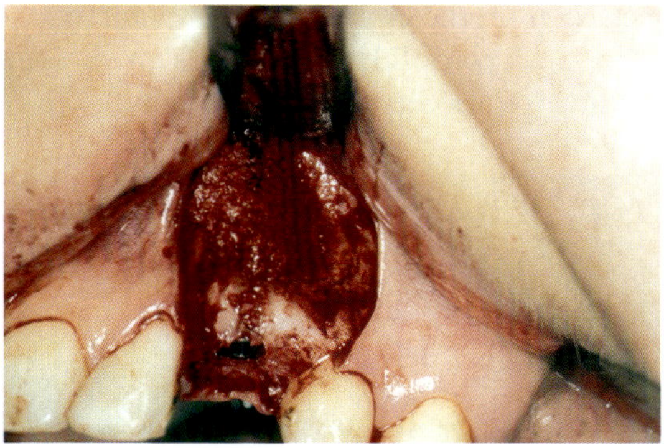

**Figure 4.7** Exposed threads covered with bone graft from BoneTrap™.

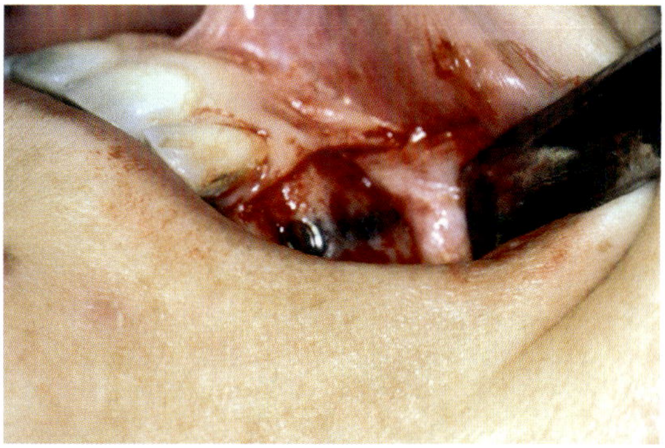

**Figure 4.8** Thin bone lamellae now covering the fixture after four to five months healing.

## 4.2 Minor bone graft in block form

In the majority of cases, onlay block grafts of cortical bone are indicated where there is a need to improve the width of the thin alveolar process or to increase the height in localized defects. Minor onlay grafts used to increase width are often placed buccally on the crest (buccal onlays) and secured with titanium plate screws. Cortical bone is best used as onlay while particulated bone can be used as a 'filler' around the onlay bone. It is also recommended to drill small holes with a round bur to stimulate bleeding and thus improve eventual healing. Bone grafts of this type should be left to heal for at least four to five months, if not six months, due to the cortical character of the graft.

Implants can be placed simultaneously but it is also advisable to let the bone heal first before implant insertion, especially if the original crest is too thin for implant site preparation. It is essential to obtain very good closure of the flap in order not to contaminate the bone graft

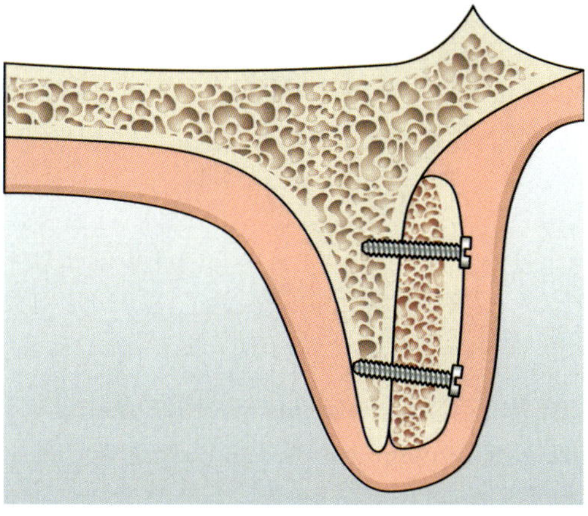

**Figure 4.9** Minor block bone graft.

material with saliva and bacteria from the oral cavity. If implant installation is made too early, before graft consolidation, there is an obvious risk that the onlay may split away from the underlying bone.

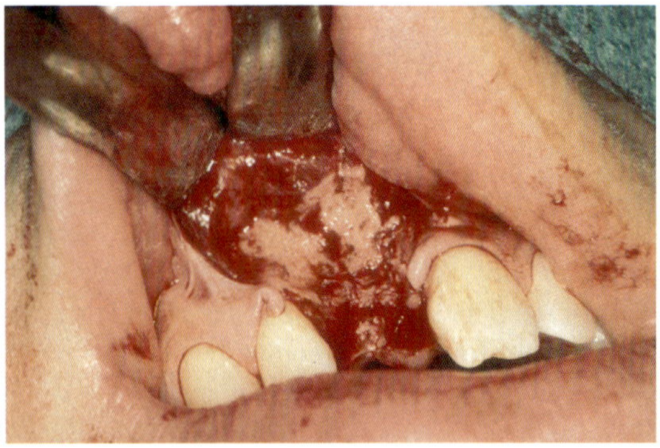

**Figure 4.10** Bone deficiency in a case of aplasia.

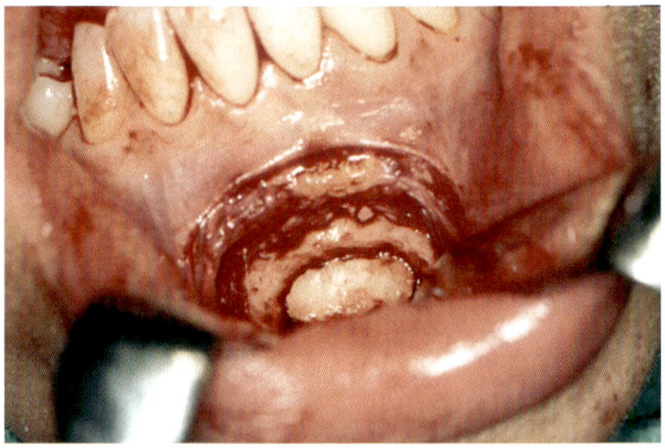

**Figure 4.11** A small circular bone graft is taken from the chin.

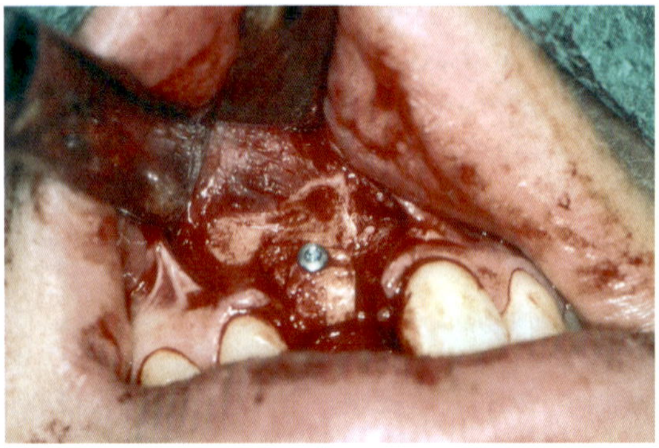

**Figure 4.12** The graft is modelled and secured with a plate screw.

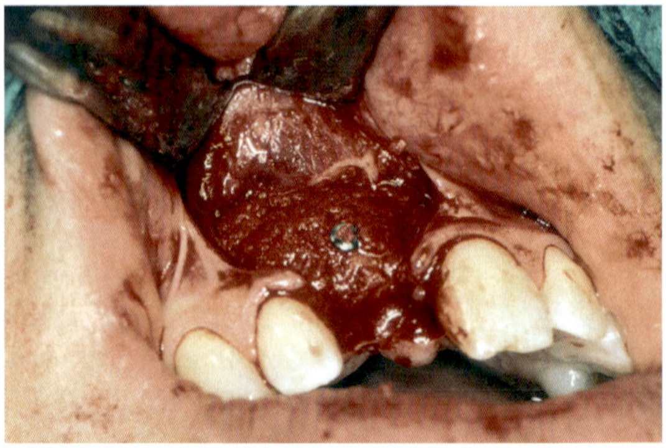

**Figure 4.13** Bone material from BoneTrap™ is packed around the onlay graft.

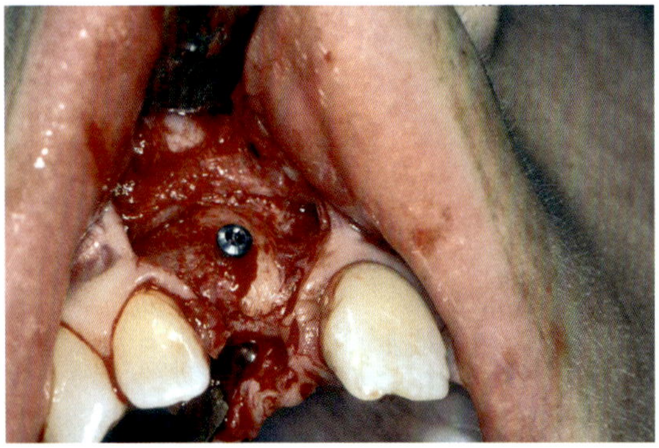

**Figure 4.14** Bone healing after five months. The graft is integrated with only minor resorption.

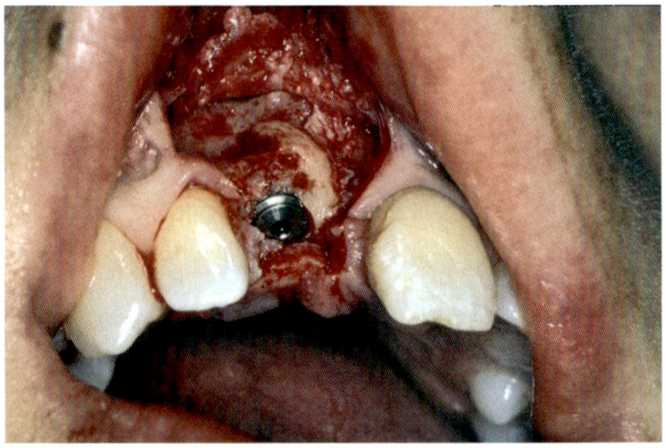

**Figure 4.15** Implant installed in the grafted bone.

## 4.3 Major onlay bone grafts in block form

Indications for larger block bone grafts are of course edentulous maxillae or almost edentulous maxillae with severe bone deficiency. In these cases the bone graft should improve the height and width of the alveolar process and enable appropriate implant positioning. It is important to use a flap technique which does not jeopardize healing of such a large bone graft volume. Also of importance is tension-free closure of the flap. Usually for this amount of bone graft the only possible harvesting site is the iliac crest. For a whole maxilla you can use a whole block or divide it in two or three pieces. The blocks are trimmed to fit onto the alveolar process as tightly as possible. The graft bed is prepared by drilling a large number of small holes using a round bur to stimulate healing. The graft material can be connected to the residual bone crest either by use of titanium plate screws or by the implants.

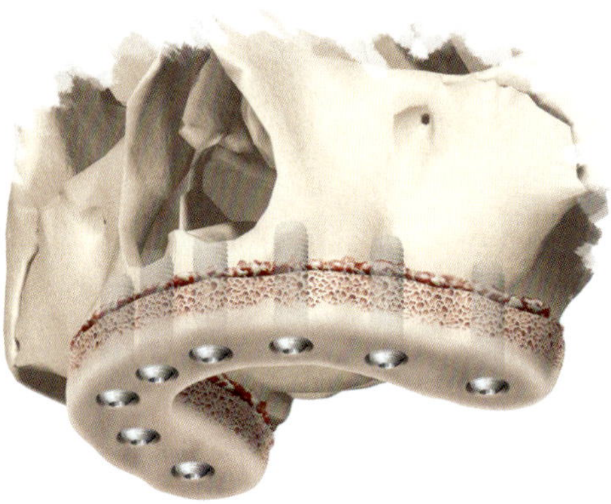

**Figure 4.16** Onlay bone grafting.

Graft healing is recommended for at least six months. If implants are installed in a second phase, healing of the implants should also be around six months. You can gain time by placing implants simultaneously but one can risk loss of implants if complications occur during the healing phase. It has also been shown that implant integration takes a considerably longer time in fresh block bone graft. Although the success rate of using bone blocks for onlay grafts in long-term follow-up has been shown to be around 70–80%, the use of this technique has decreased with time as other methods have become available.

As always, careful prosthetic loading both during healing and within the first six to twelve months after abutment connection is a prerequisite for the success of the final outcome. However, long-term follow-up has shown that there is a remarkably good preservation of the bone volume.

Onlay grafting methods do have their place in the rehabilitation of implant patients especially if there are large bony defects in the alveolar process or localized traumatic loss of part of the buccal or lingual ridge. It is the definitive treatment of choice where the ridge has a good height but is lacking in width. The most important requirements when undertaking major onlay grafting, which cannot be stressed too much, are the need for tight closure of the flap over the grafted region but with no tension in the flap, which would jeopardize vascularization and thus the healing process. With major bone blocks it is also necessary to have a flap of sufficient thickness. Large amounts of bone and bone blocks have to be harvested from the iliac crest but smaller amounts can be obtained from the mandibular symphysis or the mandibular angle region.

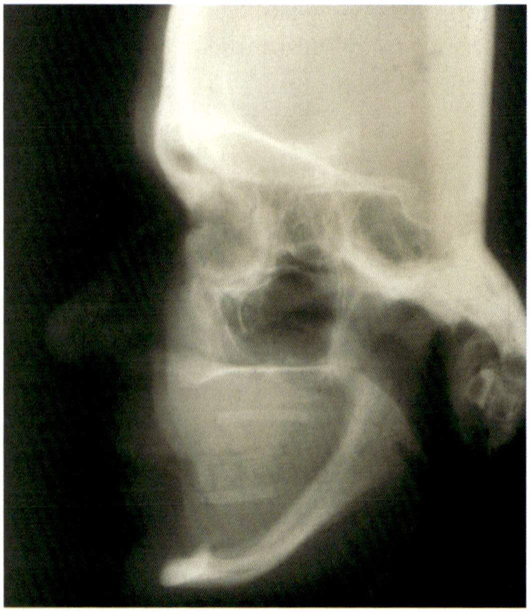

**Figure 4.17** Patient with severely resorbed maxilla.

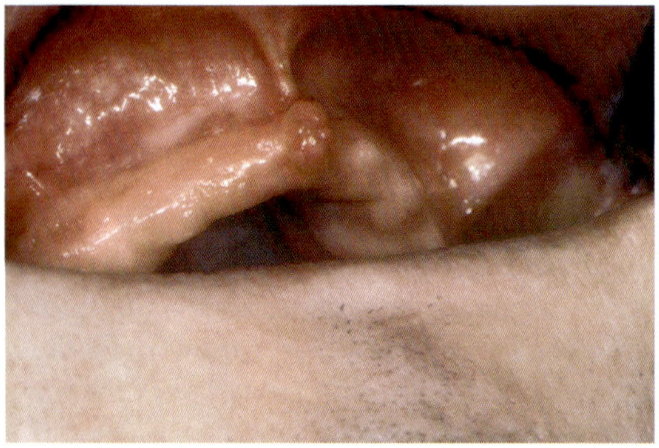

**Figure 4.18** Vestibular incision prior to onlay block grafting of the whole maxilla.

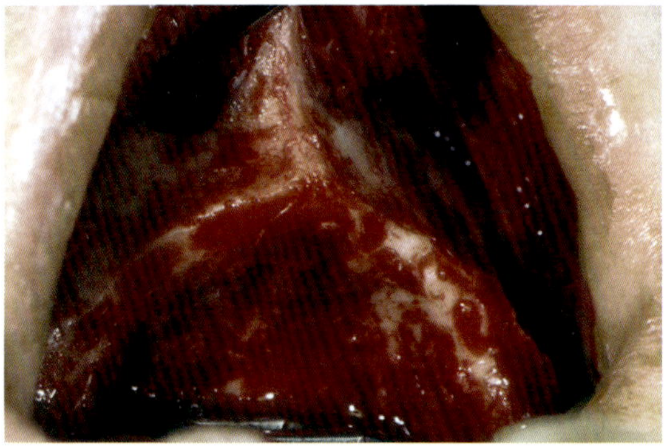

**Figure 4.19** The bony maxilla is exposed and the nasal mucosa lifted carefully.

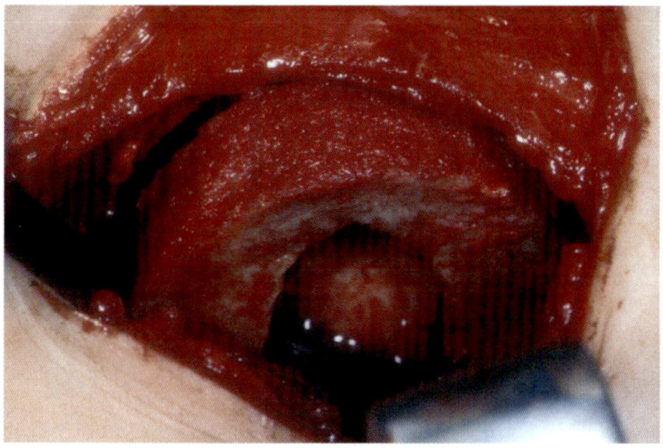

**Figure 4.20** Horseshoe shaped graft is obtained from the iliac bone below the iliac crest.

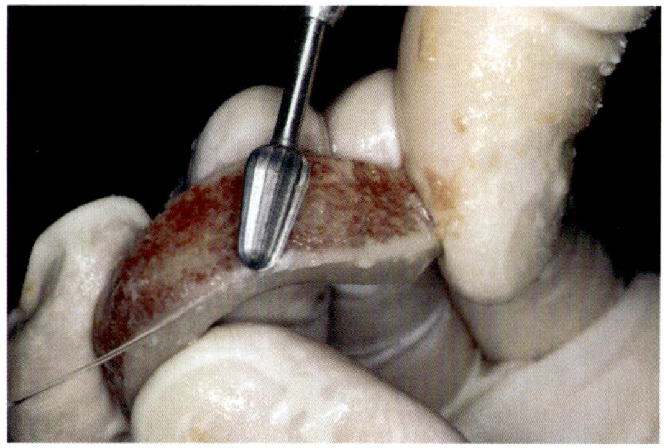

**Figure 4.21** The bone graft is modeled to fit onto the alveolar crest in all directions.

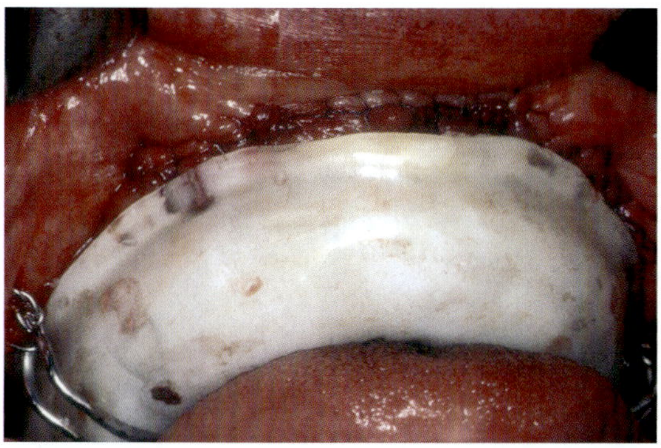

**Figure 4.22** Light compression of the soft tissue by the acrylic stent connected to the zygoma.

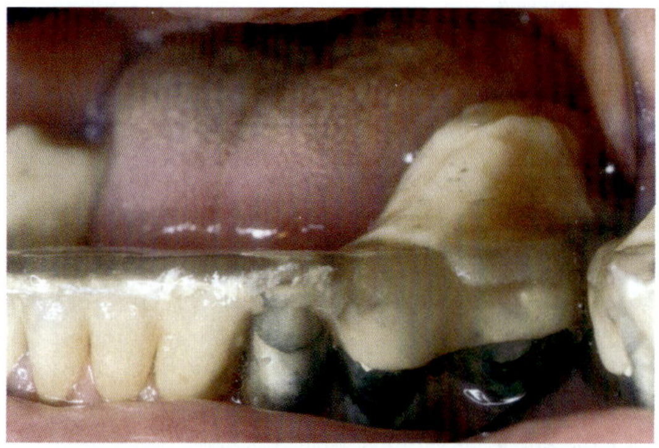

**Figure 4.23** Acrylic wafer with posterior extension to avoid trauma to the grafted region.

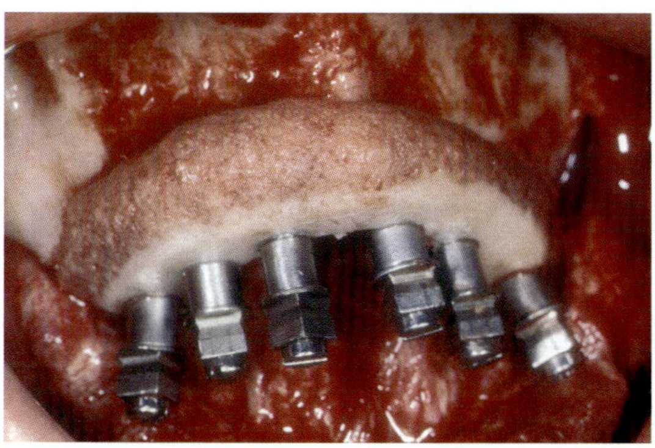

**Figure 4.24** The onlay bone graft is connected to the alveolar crest by simultaneous insertion of the implant screws.

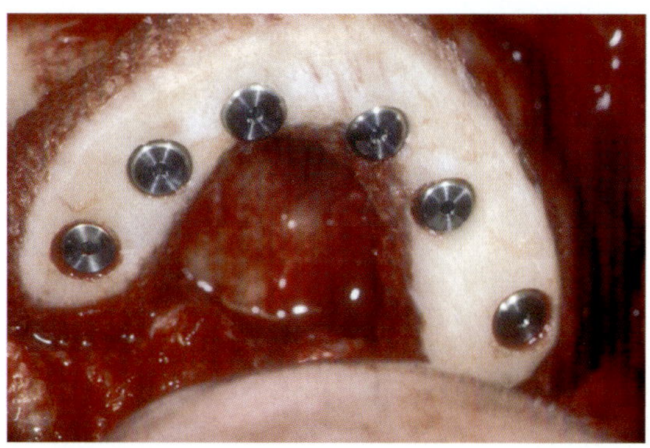

**Figure 4.25** Careful attention is taken to remove all sharp edges of the graft.

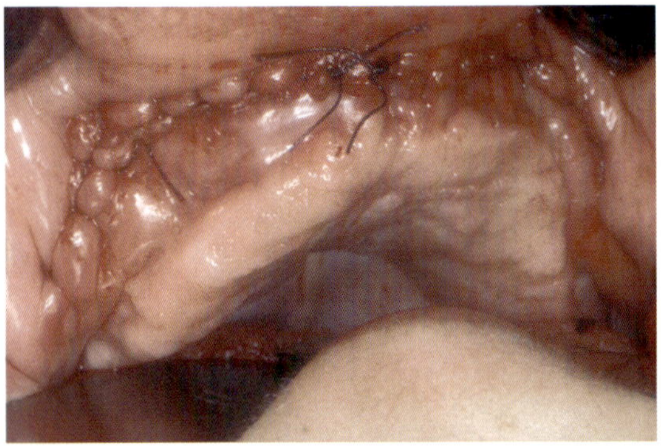

**Figure 4.26** The incision is closed with continuous suturing.

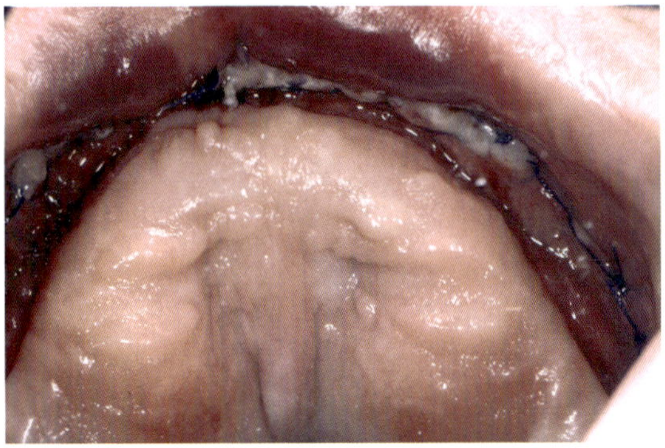

**Figure 4.27** Soft tissue healing after ten days.

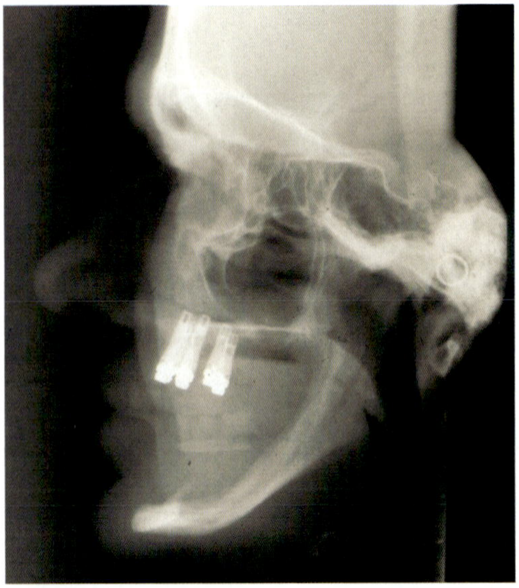

**Figure 4.28** Implants in place in the upper jaw.

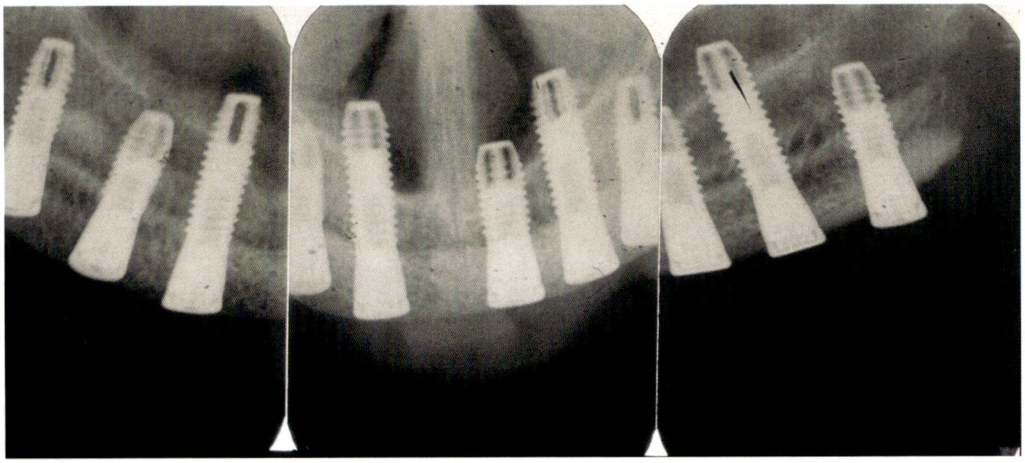

**Figure 4.29** Radiograph of bone graft and implants.

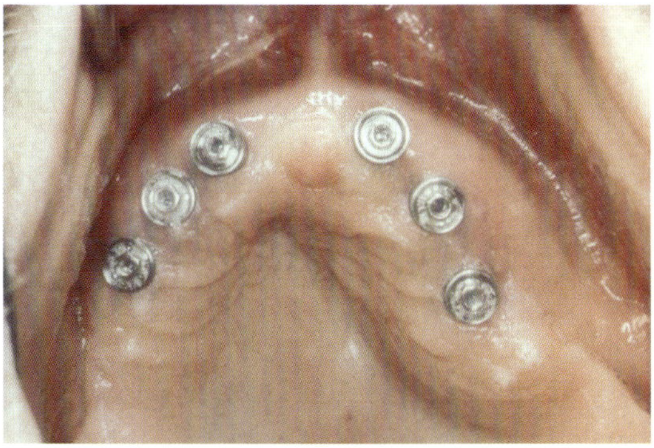

**Figure 4.30** Bone graft and implants after healing for six months.

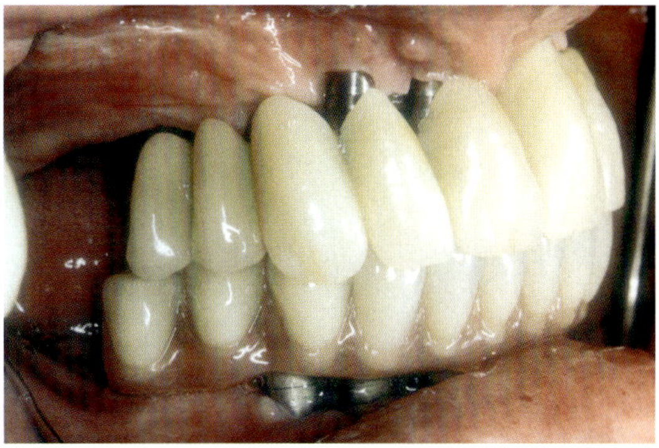

**Figure 4.31** Prosthetic reconstruction after one year.

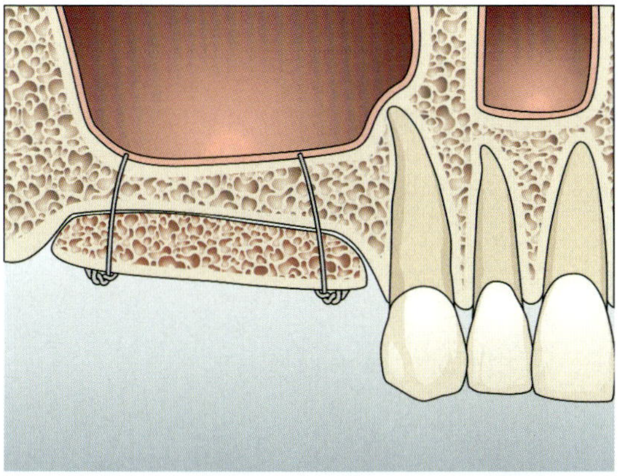

**Figure 4.32** Graft with osteosutures.

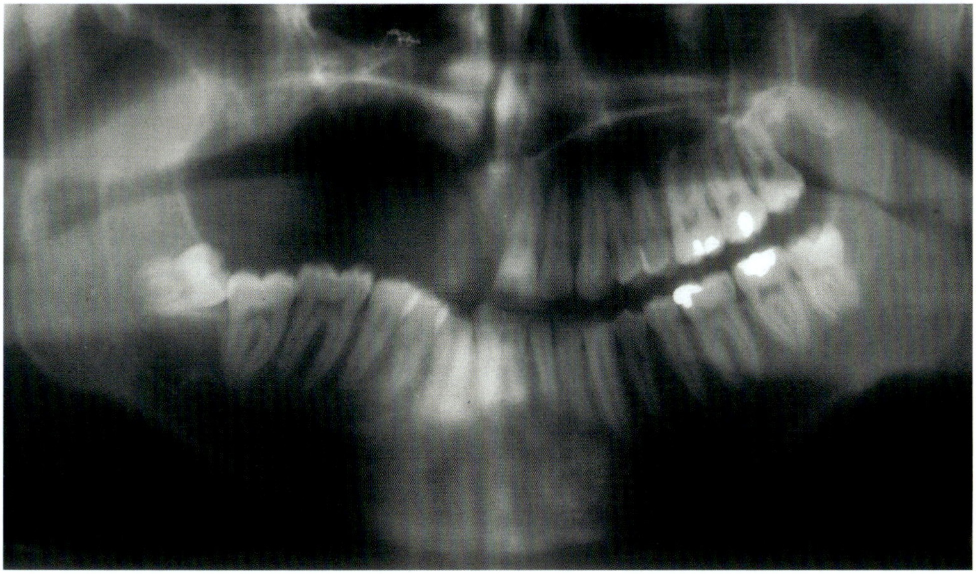

**Figure 4.33** A defect in the alveolar process in the right posterior maxilla after trauma.

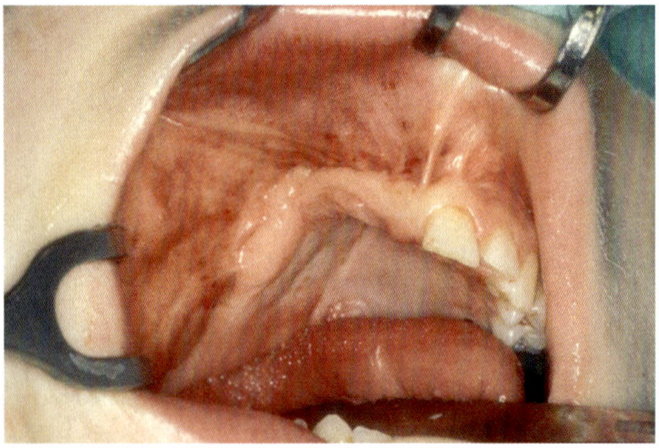

**Figure 4.34** The clinical situation.

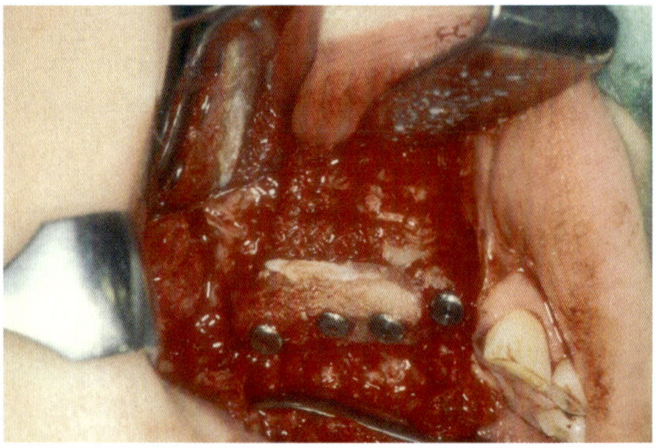

**Figure 4.35** Onlay block graft from the hip connected to the residual bone by means of the implants.

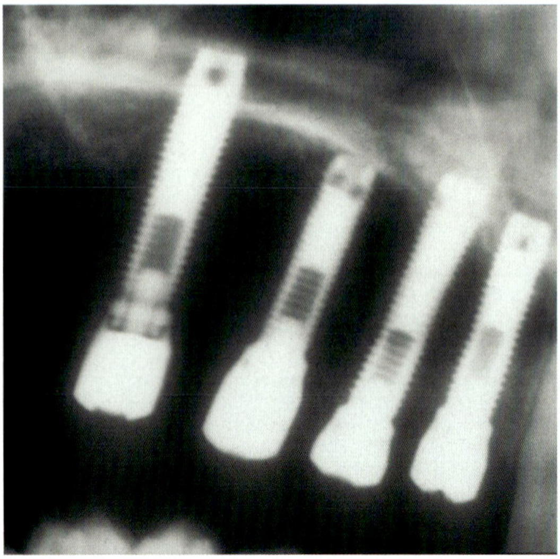

**Figure 4.36** Postoperative radiograph showing demineralized bone graft. The implants seem to be without support.

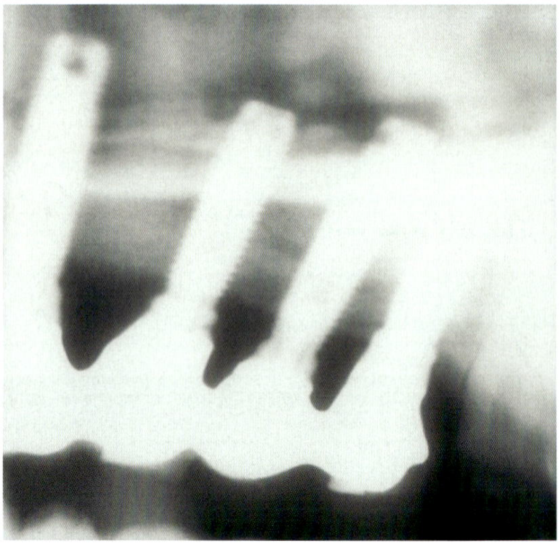

**Figure 4.37** One year later the bone graft contour is clearly visible.

## 4.4 To be mentioned

Widening of a thin, high crest can also be achieved by splitting the crest in the middle and placing graft material in between the buccal and lingual cortical plates. The problem is that it demands two cortical layers and intermediate cancellous bone otherwise there is a risk of crest fracture. If there is a thick enough crest to consist of two cortical plates and intermediate cancellous bone it is often possible to install a fixture.

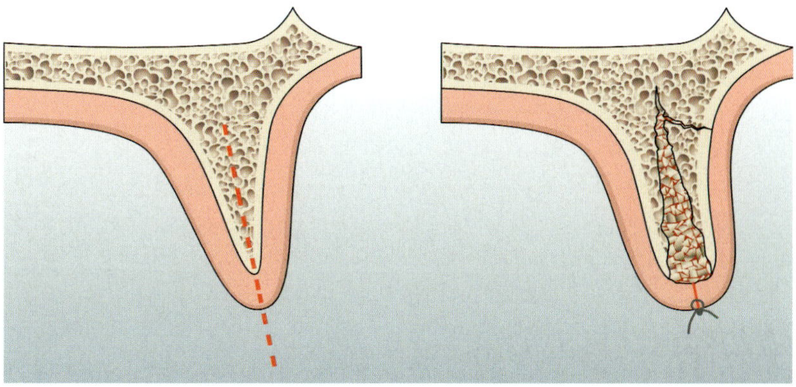

**Figure 4.38** Split crest technique for the alveolar process.

# 5 Inlay Bone Grafting

## 5.1 Nasal inlay grafting

If it is necessary to increase bone volume in the subnasal area for placement of implants and/or when combined with sinus lifting procedures, you may use the concavity just posterior to the bony nostril. By careful blunt dissection, the nasal mucosa can be lifted from the bony floor of the cavity to obtain a pocket big enough for a small bone graft. By this method you may gain 3–5 mm of bone. There is normally no need for fixation of the graft since the nasal mucosa will compress the graft towards the nasal floor. Healing time is as with onlay grafts i.e. about 4–5 months, but this may be somewhat longer if the bone is mainly cortical.

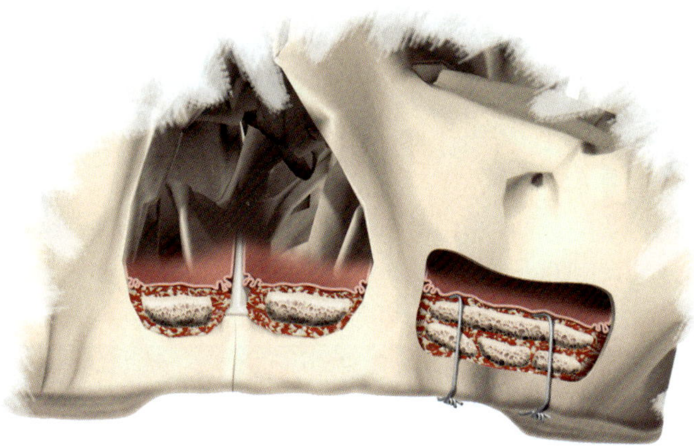

**Figure 5.1** Inlay bone grafting.

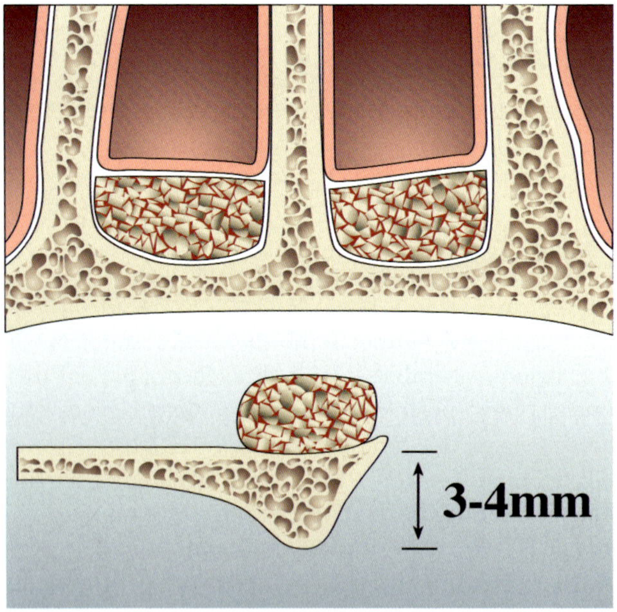


**Figure 5.2** Nasal inlays.

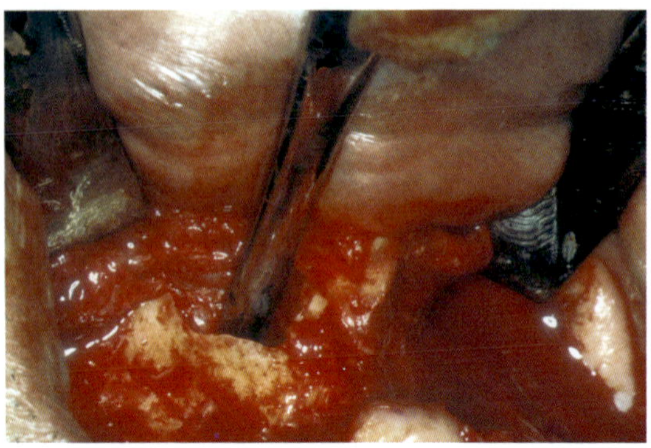

**Figure 5.3** The nasal mucosa in the nasal aperture is carefully lifted.

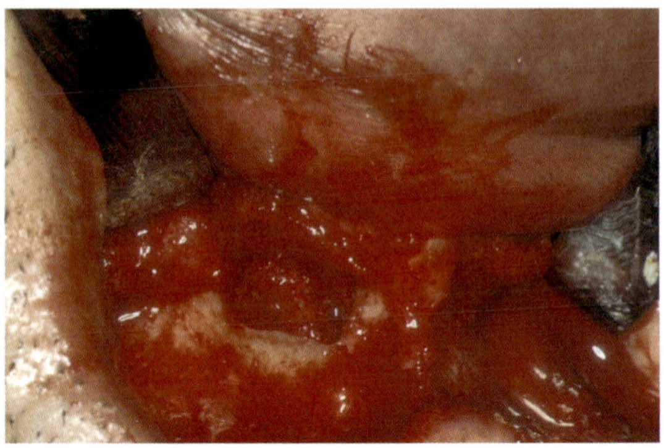

**Figure 5.4** Bone graft is pressed into the nasal cavity below the nasal mucosa.

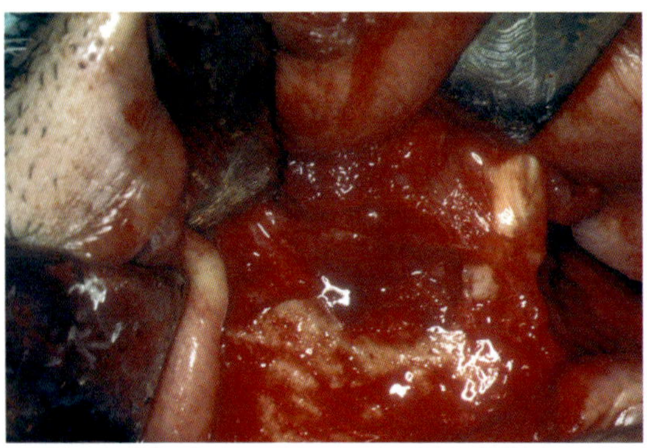

**Figure 5.5** The bony height of the alveolar process increased by 5–6 mm.

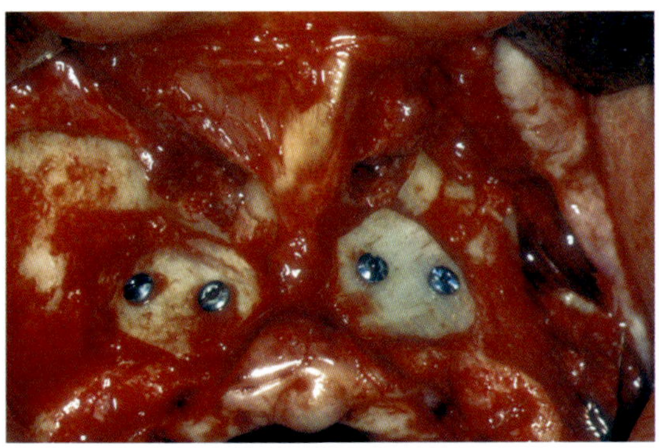

**Figure 5.6** The nasal inlays combined with onlay grafts on the thin alveolar crest.

## 5.2 Maxillary sinus grafting (sinus lifting)

Implant treatments of the edentulous posterior maxilla occasionally meet with problems due to the lack of bone volume beneath the maxillary sinus cavity. Resorption of the alveolar process after loss of posterior teeth support can proceed either from the oral side or by expansion of the sinus cavity into the alveolar process, or both. Resorption from loading by partial dentures can reduce the remaining alveolar process and minimize the bone volume available for implants. Depending on esthetic demands it may be necessary to carry out an augmentation of the ridge by onlay grafting. However, in the majority of cases, grafting of the maxillary sinus is preferred with placement of the graft into the intrasinus space occupying the alveolar process.

One of the prerequisites when intruding into the sinus cavity is to maintain the integrity of the sinus membrane (mucosa). It is well known that foreign particles that pass into the maxillary sinus cavity will, in most cases, cause an inflammatory reaction and thus loss of the grafting material and, in the case of simultaneous placement of both bone graft and implants, all graft material and implants can fail. The condition of the maxillary sinus with regard to chronic inflammation must of course be considered before starting a sinus lifting procedure. It may sometimes be impossible to avoid perforating the mucosa. If perforation does occur, it is of the utmost importance to secure the bone graft in order to avoid mobility and dislocation of the graft material into the sinus cavity. An understanding and respect for the maxillary sinus cavity as a closed, ventilated circuit, with only a narrow passage to the nose via the osteum, must be borne in mind when performing sinus lifting procedures. Because of the limited drainage from the sinus cavity it is also recommended to avoid formation of small spaces where it may be difficult to eliminate blood and remnants of debris. It is recommended that the sinus cavity be augmented in such a way as not to produce an irregular internal contour of the sinus floor.

Fixation of block graft material in cases where there is insufficient stability of the graft is obtained either by wire osteosynthesis or by titanium plate screws. The most frequently used graft material is autologous bone material either from the iliac crest, the tibia, mandibular symphysis region, the mandibular angle or maxillary tuberosity. The graft material may consist of both cortical and cancellous bone and may also be milled to form a particulated bone material. This bone material can then be mixed with artificial bone material up to a 50:50 ratio without affecting the healing process and bone formation.

If only a little graft material is needed, small bone graft particles can be 'nibbled' from the neighbourhood of the surgical site. Collection of bone material during drilling of fixture sites by using the BoneTrap™

has also proven to be very efficient, with remarkably large amounts of bone powder material being collected.

The choice of graft site obviously depends on the amount of bone graft necessary for the surgical procedure. For example, if a larger amount of bone graft is needed in total maxillary grafting, the only possible graft site is the iliac crest. In unilateral sinus lifting procedures, bone grafts from the chin or mandibular angle may be sufficient for implant retention. It is yet to be determined which autologous bone graft material is best but theory suggests that the skull and jaw bones may offer a superior result, due to their similar embryologic origin. Calvarial bone is also used as a source for grafting by using the outer cortical layer from the parietal and/or occipital bones.

### 5.2.1 *Single implant procedure with local sinus lifting in a one-stage procedure*

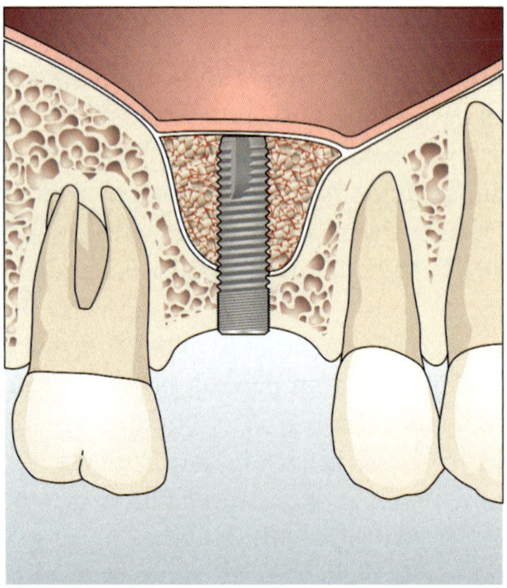

**Figure 5.7** Local sinus lift procedure.

In cases of replacement of a single premolar or molar tooth in the maxilla where the sinus cavity is close to the marginal bone, it may be necessary to increase bone volume by a sinus lifting procedure. If there is 4–5 mm of marginal bone available, it is possible to do a one-stage grafting and implant procedure. However, if the marginal bone height is below this it will be difficult to initially stabilize the implant and a two-stage procedure is recommended.

A crestal incision and conventional flap technique is used. A circular osteotomy is made in the lateral bony wall located at the inferior border of the sinus where the implant is expected to perforate the sinus floor. The bone, including an area of about 3–4 $mm^2$ is removed by a round bur and bone material is collected simultaneously with a BoneTrap™. With care it is possible to preserve the sinus membrane and push it superiorly, thereby exposing the bony sinus floor. The implant site is prepared with a conventional technique and the implant inserted, protruding upwards into the sinus recess below the membrane without perforating it. The visible part of the implant is embedded in the bone material previously collected and the incision closed. Proposed healing time is 5–6 months before loading.

Of course it is not necessary to do a sinus lifting procedure if the remaining marginal bone height is 10 mm or more.

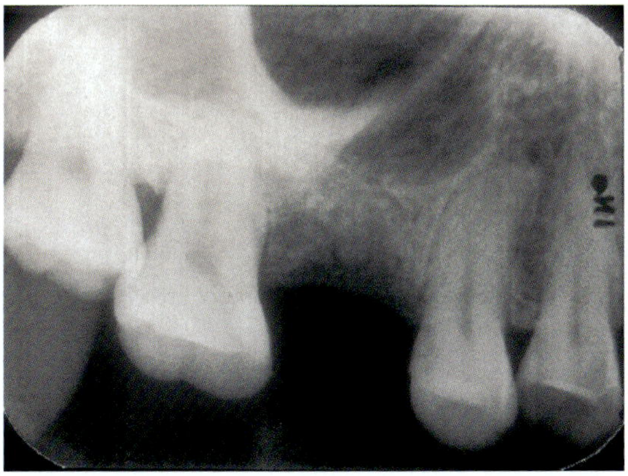

**Figure 5.8** Intraoral radiograph showing the available bone height after extraction of tooth 16.

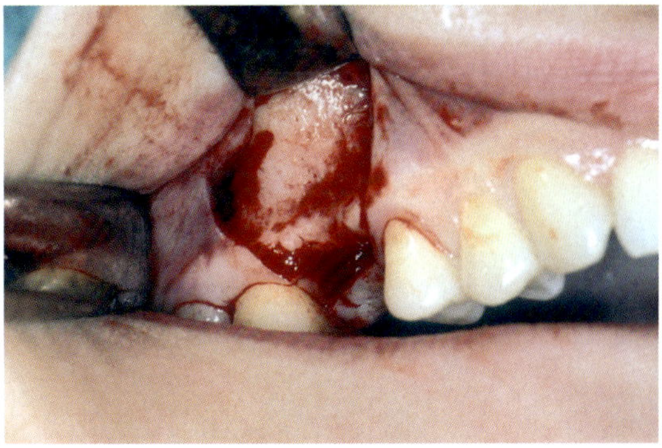

**Figure 5.9** Surgical exposure of the alveolar crest.

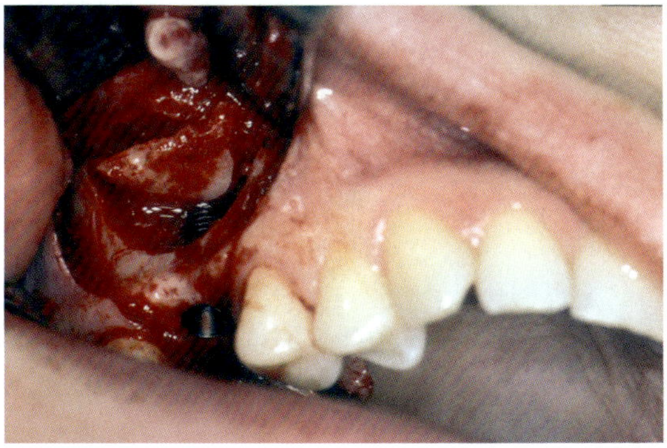

**Figure 5.10** Infracture of a bony window with simultaneous lifting of the sinus membrane and insertion of the implant.

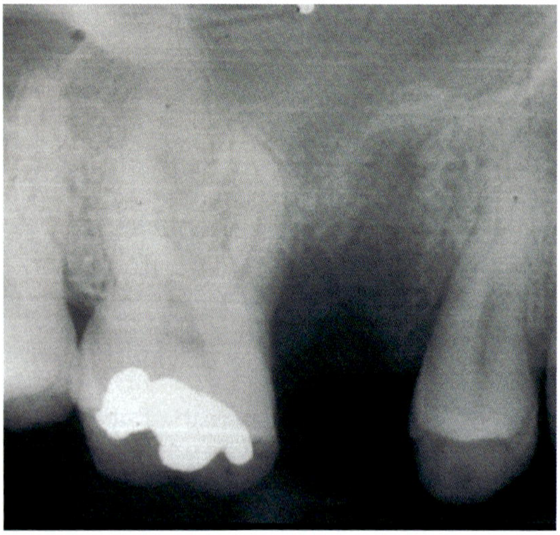

**Figure 5.11** Radiograph of extraction site after removal of second premolar.

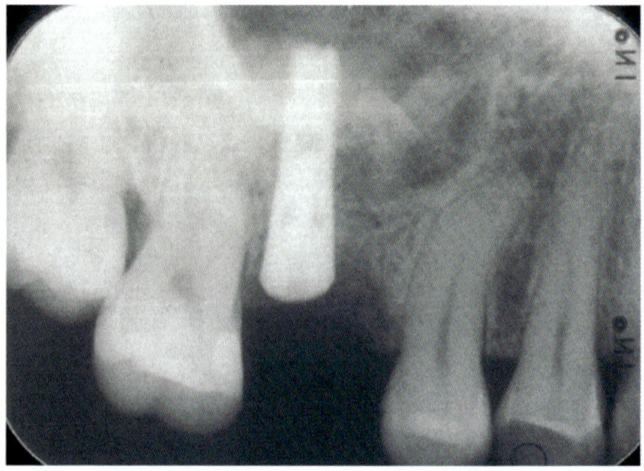

**Figure 5.12** Radiograph showing the implant in position.

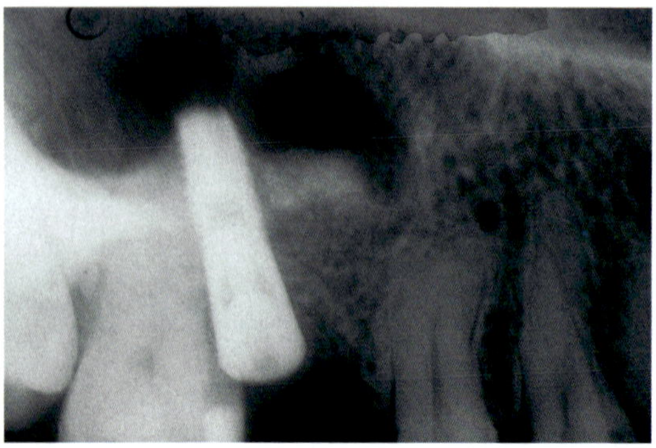

**Figure 5.13** One year postoperatively. Radiograph showing remodelling of graft material.

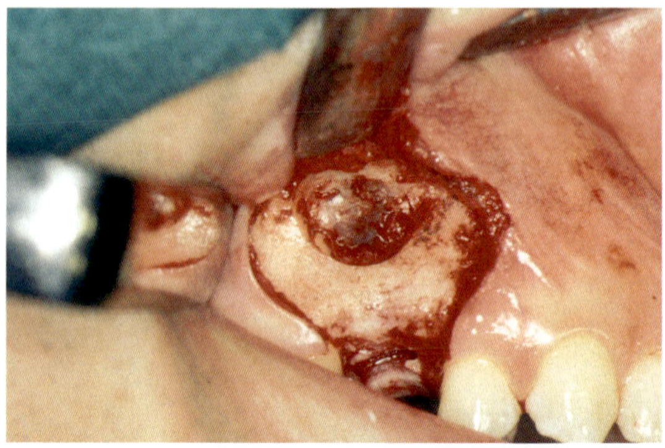

**Figure 5.14** Elevation of mucoperiosteal flap and removal of bone close to the sinus membrane.

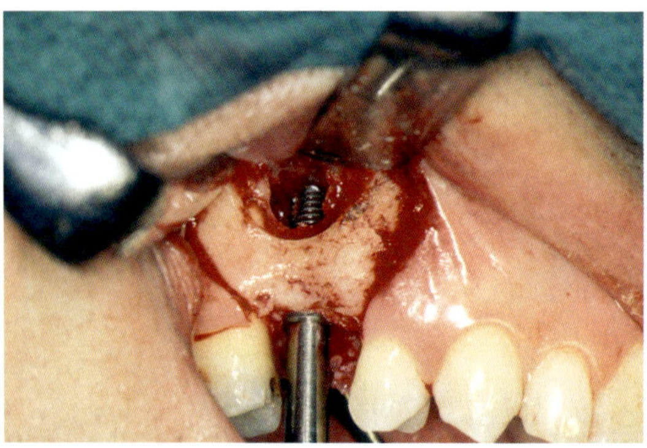

**Figure 5.15** Clinical view of implant touching and lifting the sinus membrane.

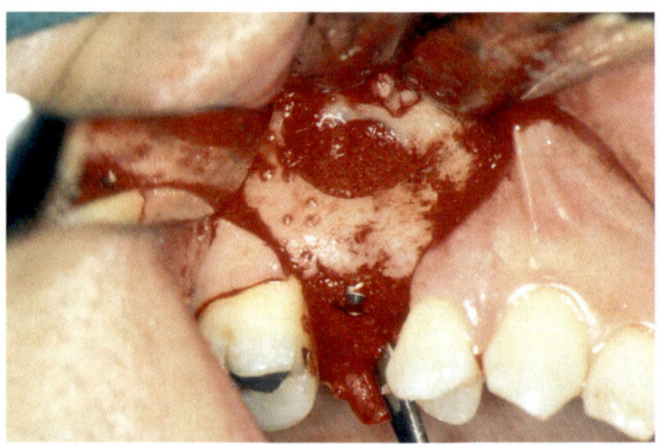

**Figure 5.16** Bone material from BoneTrap™ is packed around the exposed part of the implant.

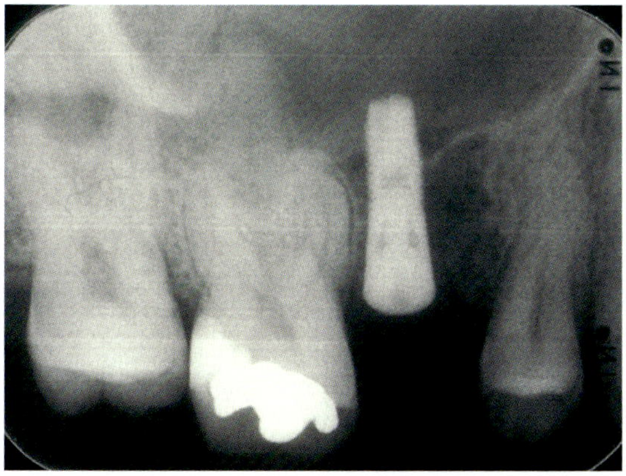

**Figure 5.17** Radiograph of implant in place where half of the implant is placed into the sinus cavity.

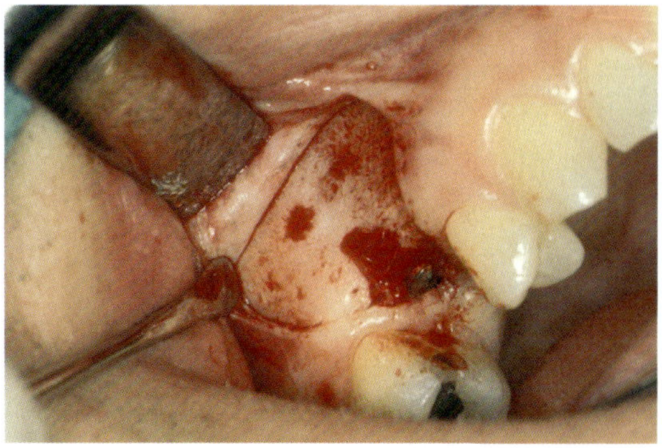

**Figure 5.18** Exposure for abutment connection four months later shows satisfactory bone healing.

### 5.2.2 *One-stage procedure with grafting and implant installation at the same time (unilateral or bilateral)*

In cases where the alveolar process of the posterior maxilla has a vertical dimension of 5–10 mm below the sinus and a width of at least 4 mm to allow primary stability of the fixtures, the implants can be placed simultaneously with the sinus bone graft.

A crestal incision is made slightly to the palatal side of the crest in order to avoid eventual rupture in the incision line during postoperative swelling. A mucoperiosteal flap is raised and the buccal aspect of the maxillary sinus exposed. A semi-circular cut is made in the lateral bony wall at the lower border of the sinus cavity with a round diamond bur. The sinus mucosa is carefully reflected superiorly. Cancellous bone is packed into the sinus recess and a cortical cancellous block placed with the cortical layer facing the sinus membrane. The block is finally pressed towards the floor while the implants are inserted through the alveolar process into the block and through the cortical plate. The bony window is positioned superior to the bone graft block, still connected with the sinus mucosa and the bone fracture line. Healing takes 6–7 months. Abutment connection is carried out according to the standard protocol.

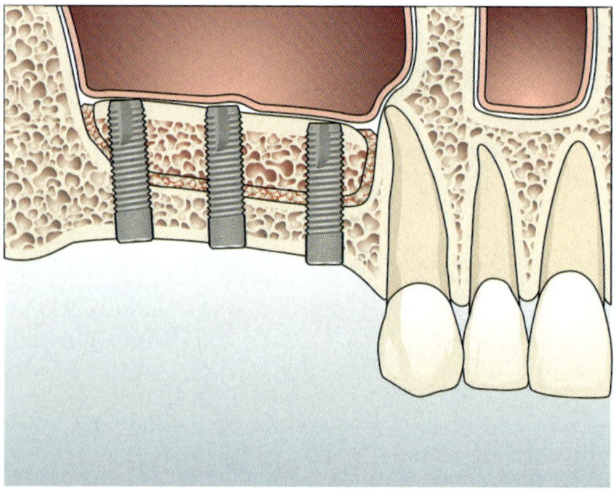

**Figure 5.19** One-stage grafting.

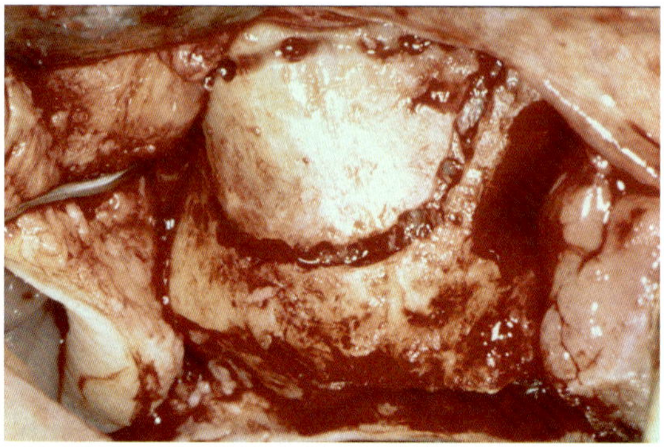

**Figure 5.20** Clinical view of posterior maxilla with elevation of mucoperiosteal flap and osteotomy performed according to the window technique using a round bur.

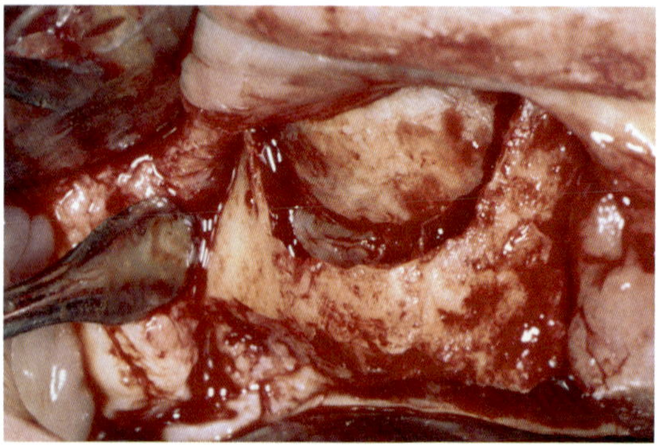

**Figure 5.21** Elevation of the sinus membrane and infracture of the bony window.

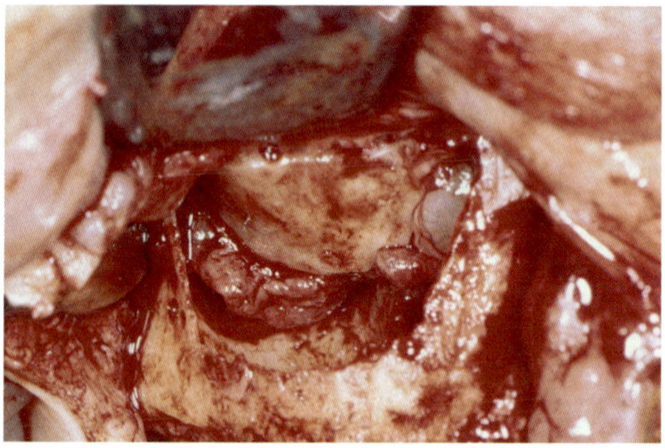

**Figure 5.22** The sinus recess is created for the bone graft by lifting the bone window and sinus mucosa.

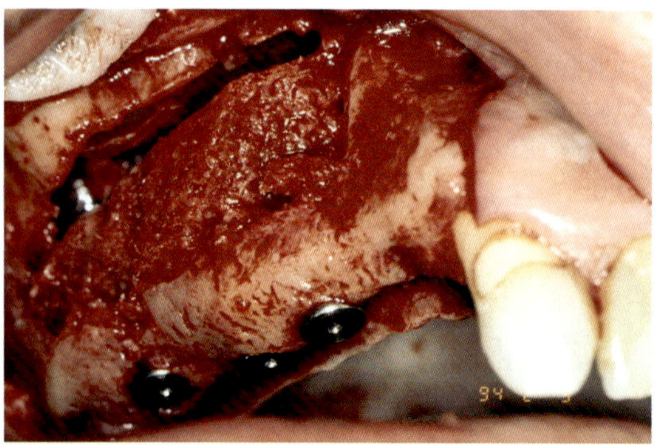

**Figure 5.23** Bone graft from iliac crest (cortical and cancellous) is positioned in the sinus recess and implants inserted.

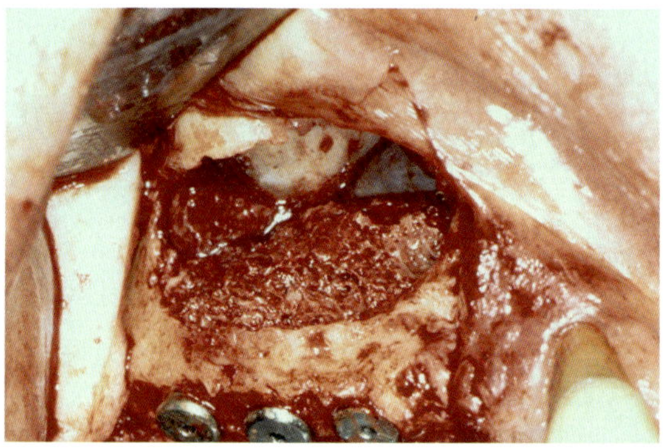

**Figure 5.24** Clinical view of bone graft and implants in relation to the sinus membrane and window.

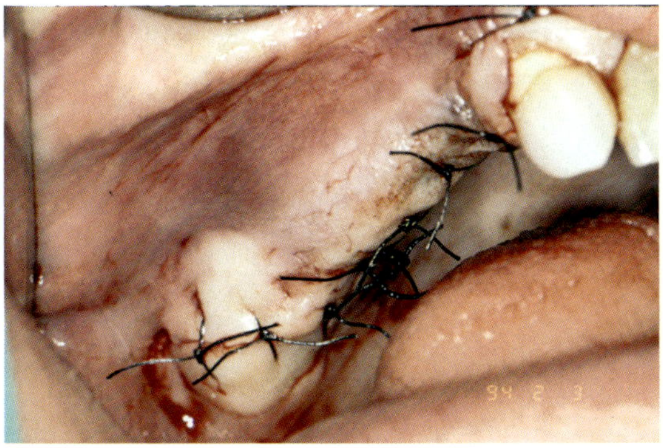

**Figure 5.25** Suturing of the flap. Note that incision line is positioned palatally of the crest.

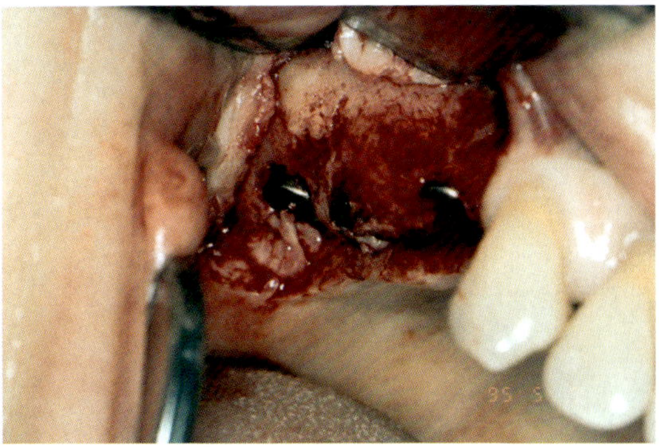

**Figure 5.26** Bone healing six months later.

### 5.2.3 *Two-stage procedure with grafting and implant installation at the staged times (unilateral or bilateral)*

Bone grafting in two stages with subsequent implant insertion is always indicated when the marginal bone height in the alveolar process is less than 5–6 mm and a width of less than 4 mm. The buccal bony window is marked and preferably kept as close as possible to the floor of the sinus cavity. In order to try to achieve a two compartment sinus cavity, it is advantageous if the buccal window is big and the superior fracture line is close to the infraorbital foramen. After penetration of the bone by a round bur or diamond bur, the sinus mucosa is carefully reflected superiorly and the window infractured into the sinus cavity. The inferior compartment creates a recess for the placement of both cancellous and cortical bone grafts. The particulated cancellous bone is positioned in the floor of the recess and the block bone above. If good stability can be achieved without wires or plate screws it is possible to omit them, however, in general a good and safe stabilization using wires or plate screws is recommended. The suggested amount of time for bone graft healing is 4–5 months. Too short a healing period may jeopardize the stability of the graft, and too long a period may allow its resorption. Five to six months should be allowed for healing of implants in the graft.

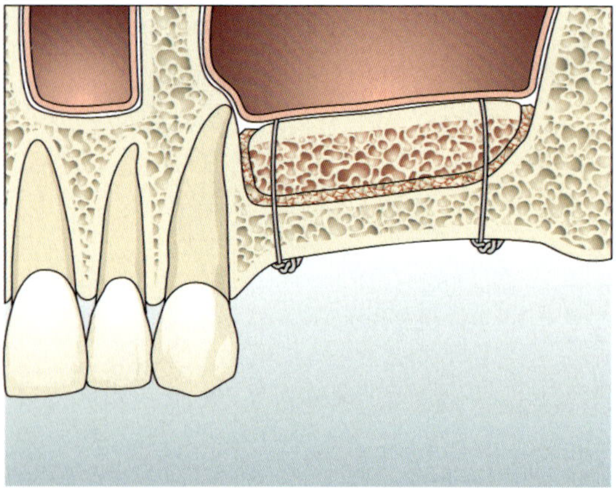

Figure 5.27 Two-stage procedure.

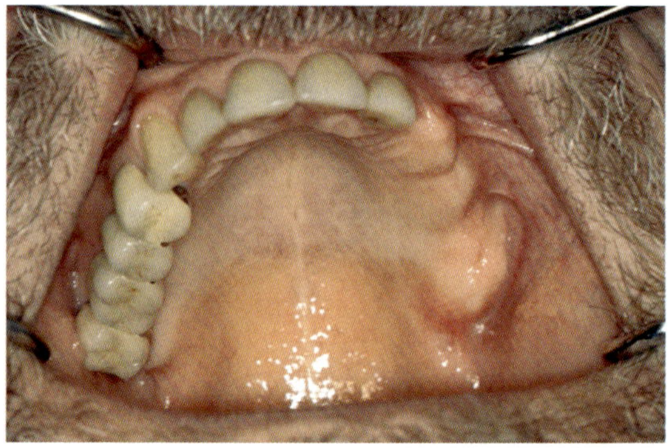

Figure 5.28 Patient with loss of teeth in the left posterior maxilla.

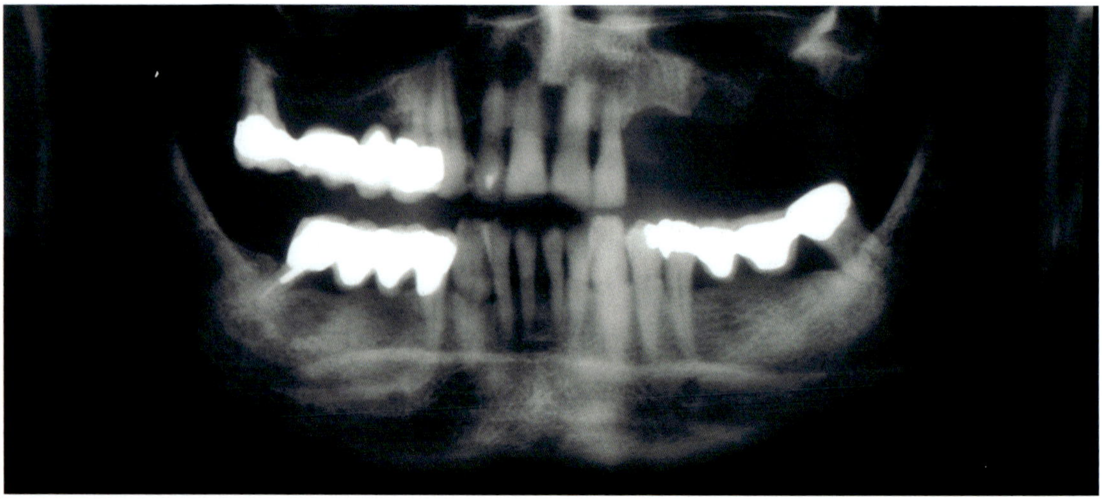

Figure 5.29 Panoramic X-ray shows inadequate bone volume beneath sinus on the left side.

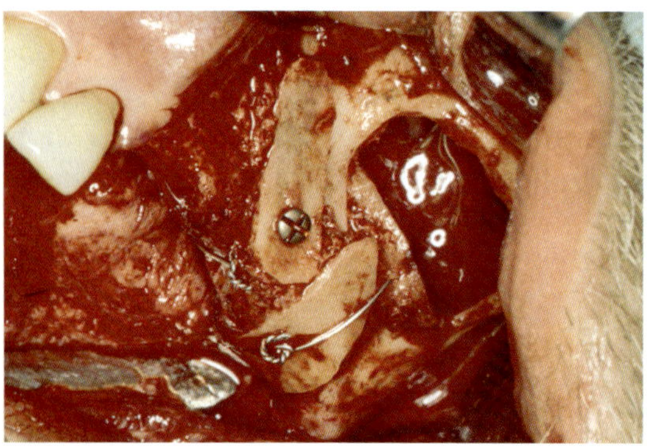

Figure 5.30 Sinus lifting with bone graft from the iliac crest. The graft is immobilized with osteosutures. The bone window is used as an onlay graft.

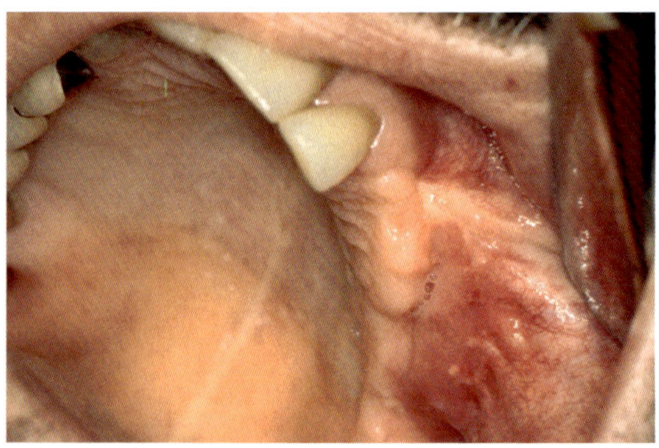

Figure 5.31 Uncomplicated healing of the soft tissues.

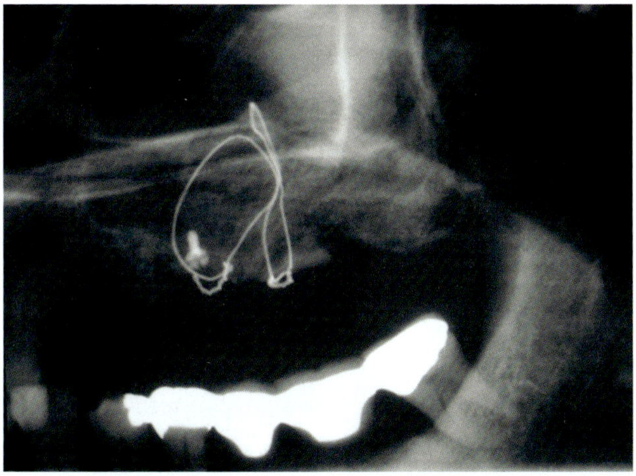

**Figure 5.32** Radiograph showing the bone graft in position.

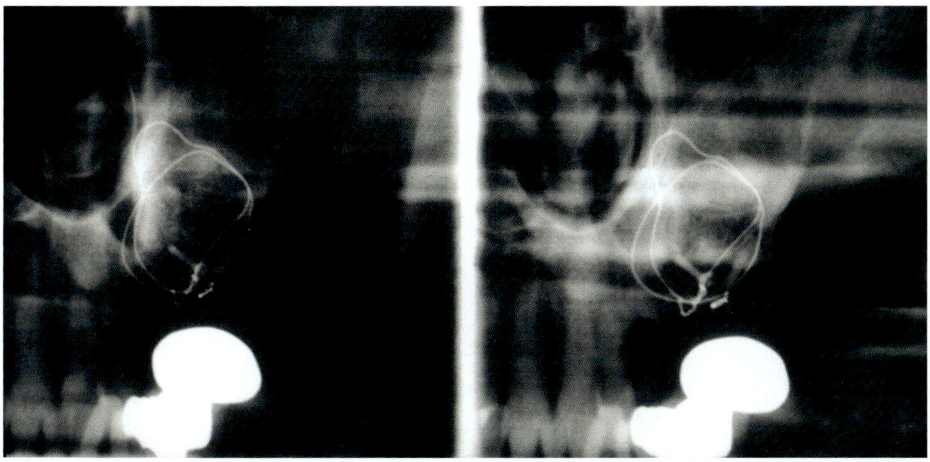

**Figure 5.33** Tomograph showing the amount of bone augmentation.

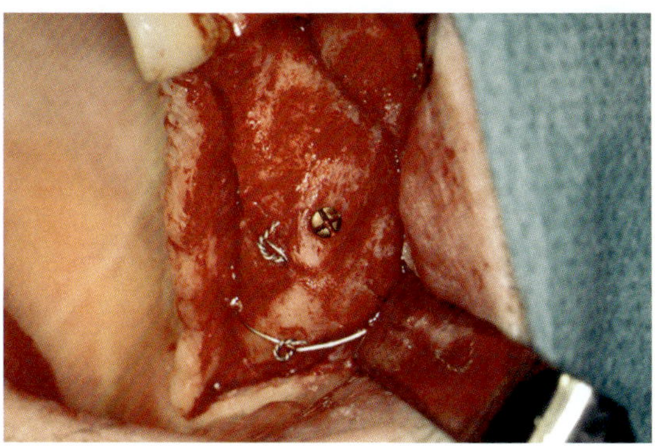

**Figure 5.34** Clinical view after four months healing.

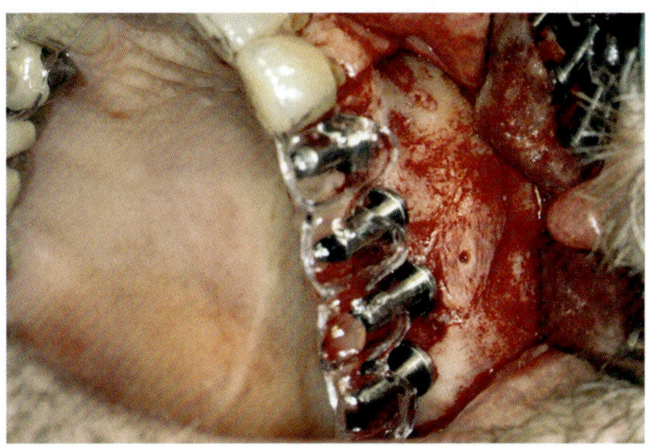

**Figure 5.35** Surgical guide for positioning of implants in the grafted bone.

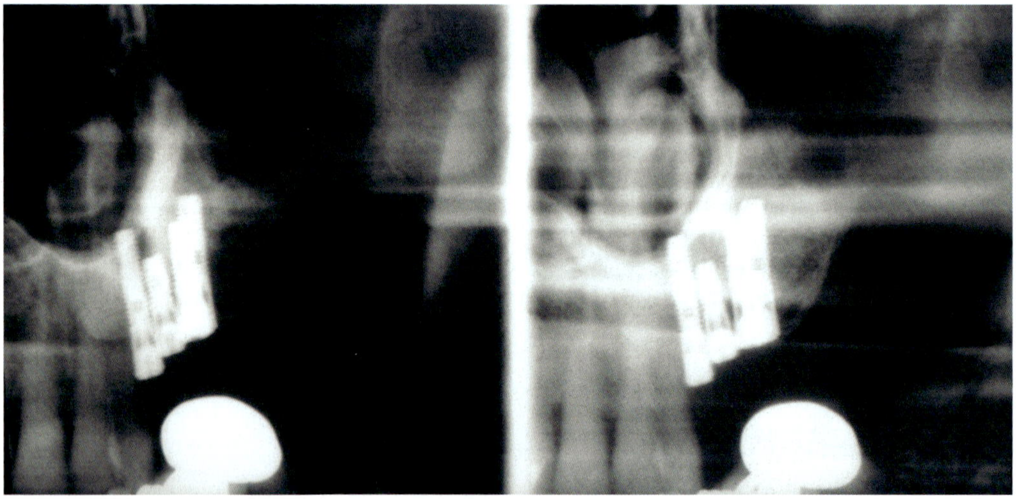

**Figure 5.36** Tomography of implants in place in the bone graft.

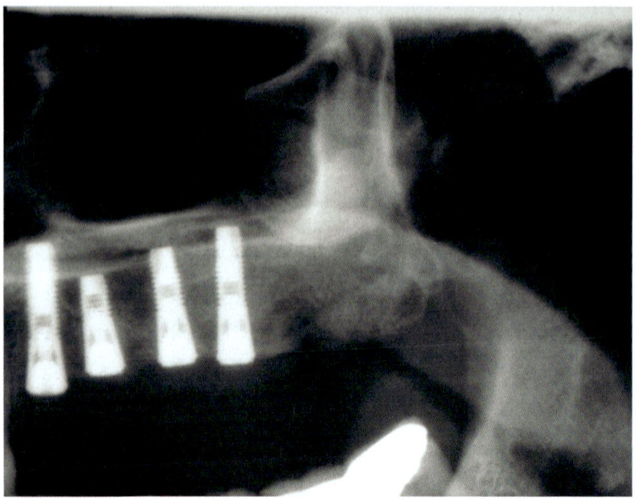

**Figure 5.37** Radiograph of the implants in the available graft material.

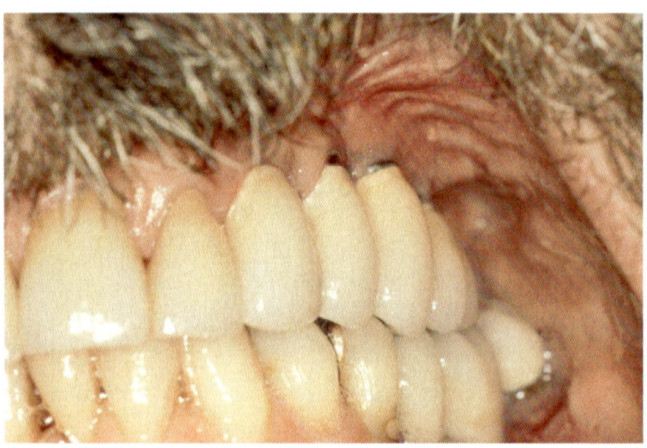

**Figure 5.38** Clinical view of definitive superstructure.

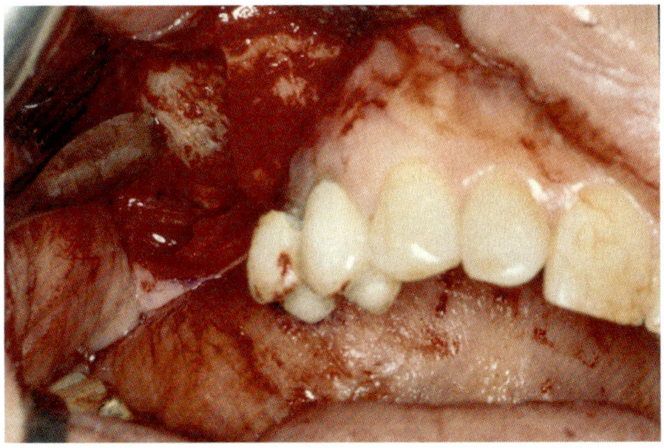

**Figure 5.39** Bone window infractured for sinus lifting procedure in the right posterior maxilla.

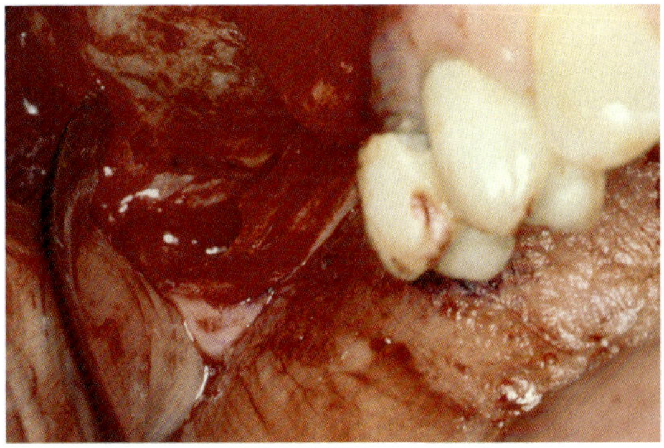

**Figure 5.40** A space is created inferior to the bone window with the sinus membrane on top of window.

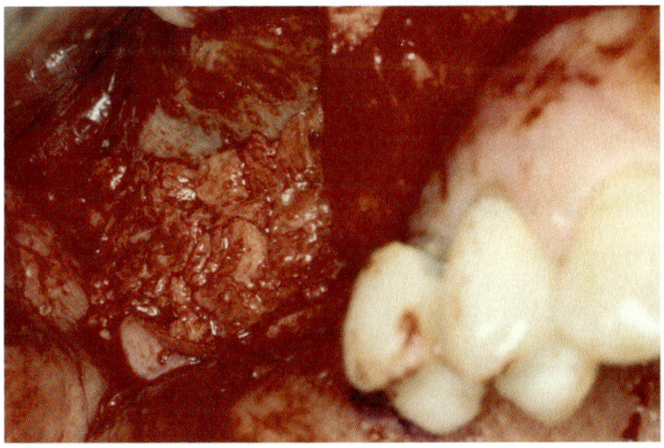

**Figure 5.41** Particulated bone graft is placed below the bony window.

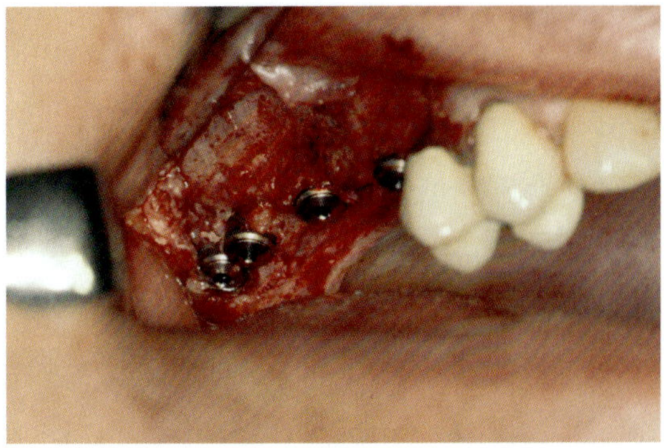

**Figure 5.42** Implants inserted after four months of healing.

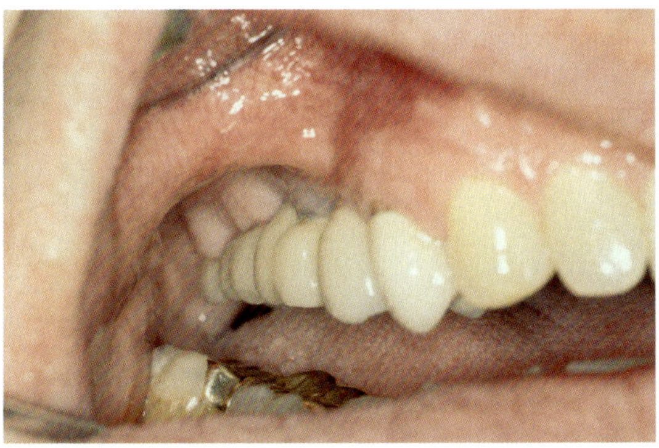

**Figure 5.43** Bridge connected to implants.

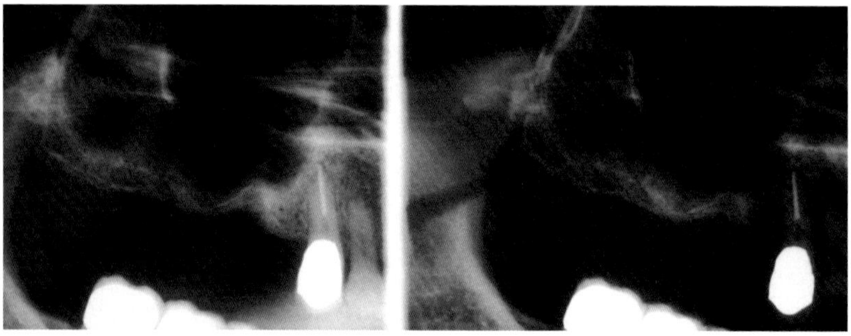

**Figure 5.44** Radiograph of right posterior maxilla showing sinus cavity occupying the alveolar process.

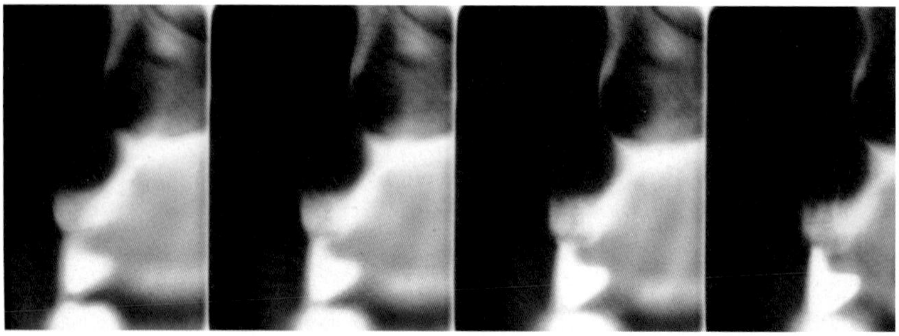

**Figure 5.45** Tomography showing the residual bone volume.

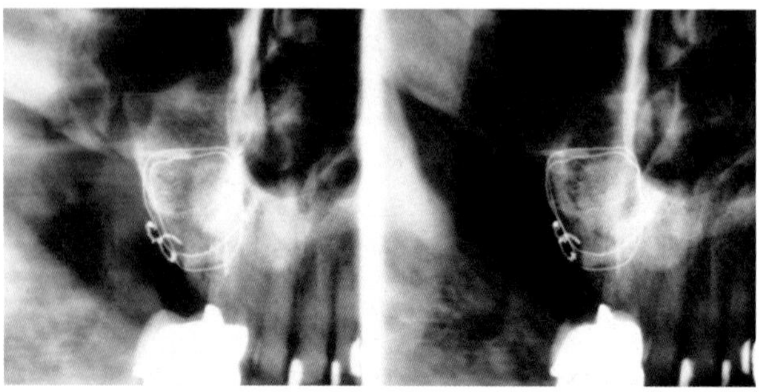

**Figure 5.46** Tomography after bone graft placement and wires.

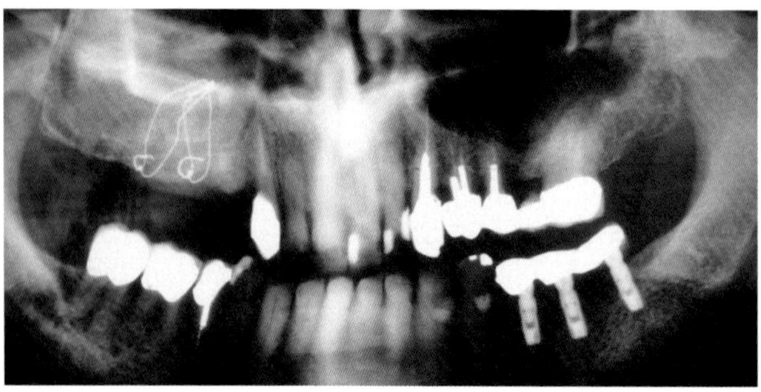

**Figure 5.47** Panoramic view showing the bone graft reconstruction of the right posterior maxilla.

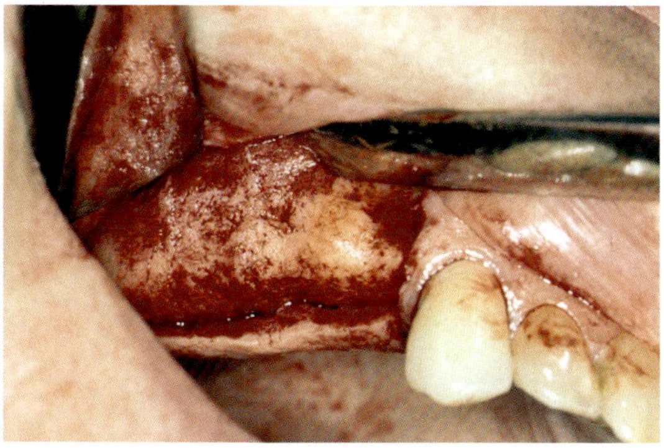

**Figure 5.48** Bony union of graft material after four months.

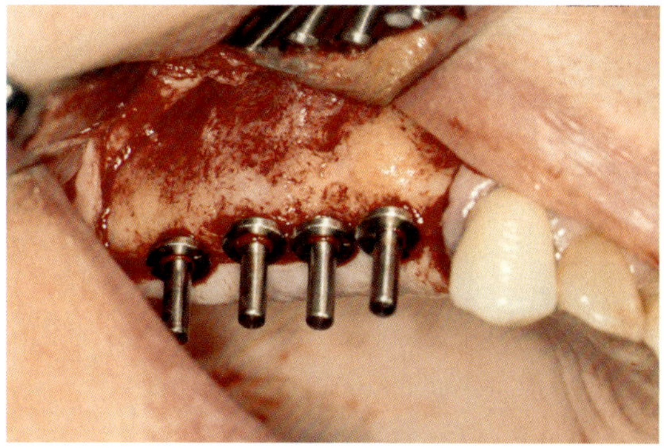

**Figure 5.49** Preparation of implant site and guide pins.

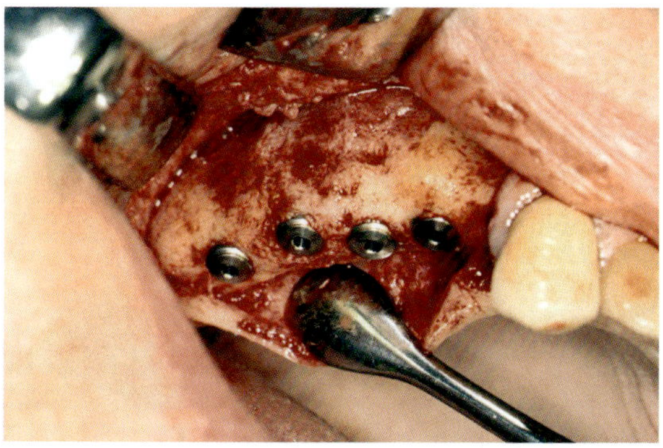

**Figure 5.50** Radiograph showing position of implants.

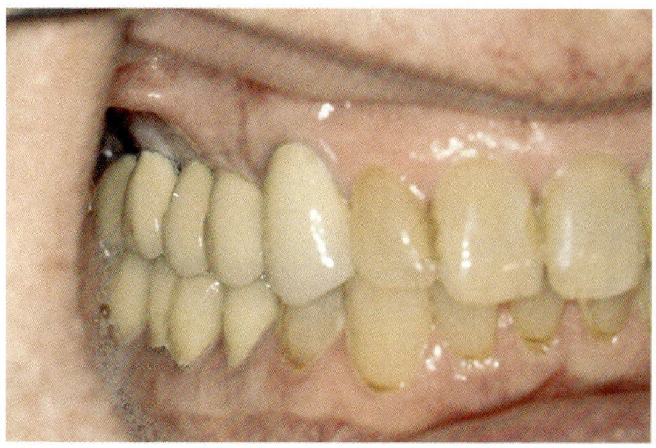

**Figure 5.51** Implants placed in grafted bone.

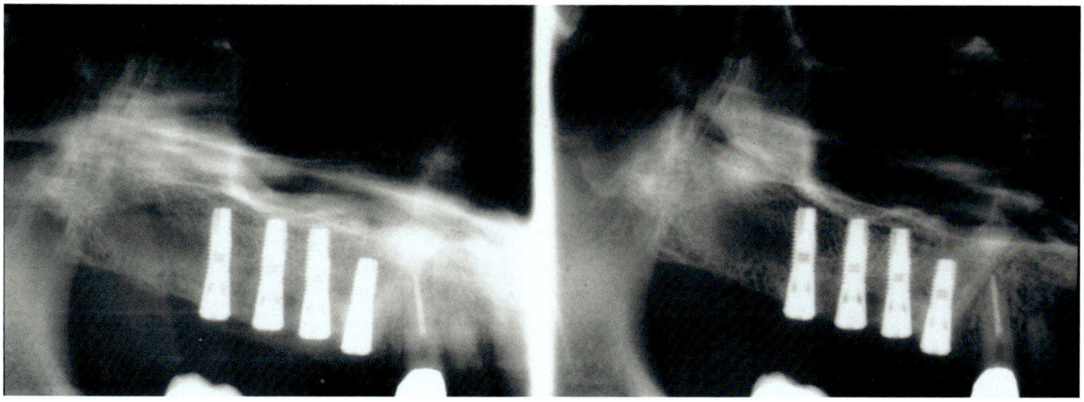

**Figure 5.52** Bridge construction on four implants.

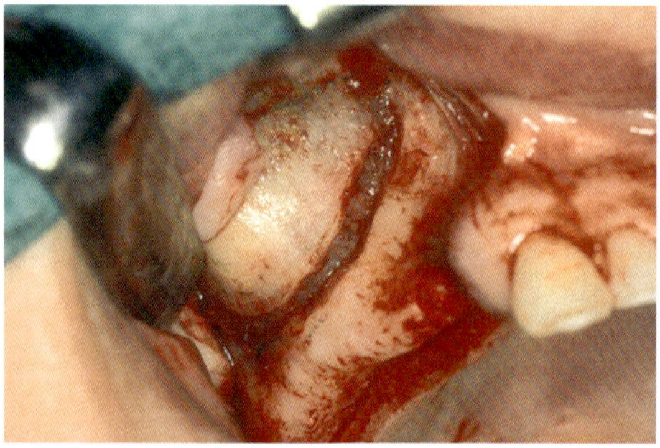

**Figure 5.53** Clinical view of bone window in right posterior maxilla.

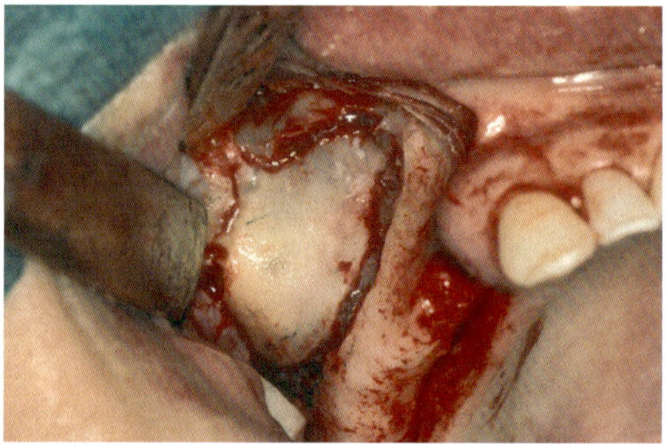

**Figure 5.54** Infracture of bone window with elevation of sinus membrane.

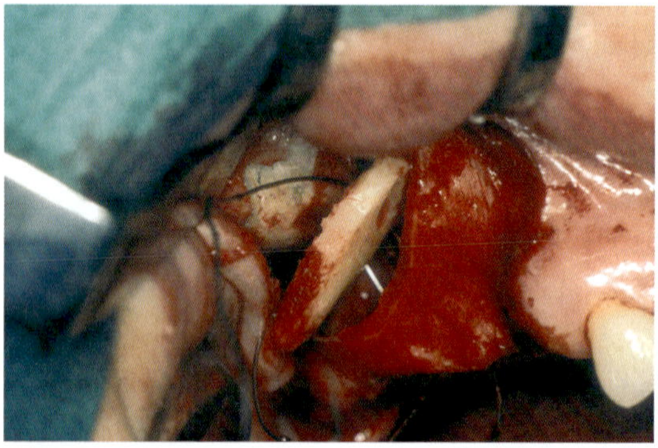

**Figure 5.55** Bone graft from the right mandibular angle (cortical) positioned below the bone window and sinus mucosa. Osteosuture is introduced around the graft material.

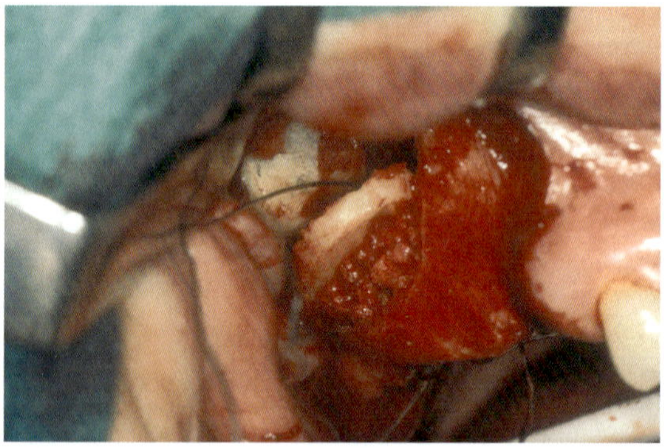

**Figure 5.56** Space below the cortical graft is filled with particulated bone.

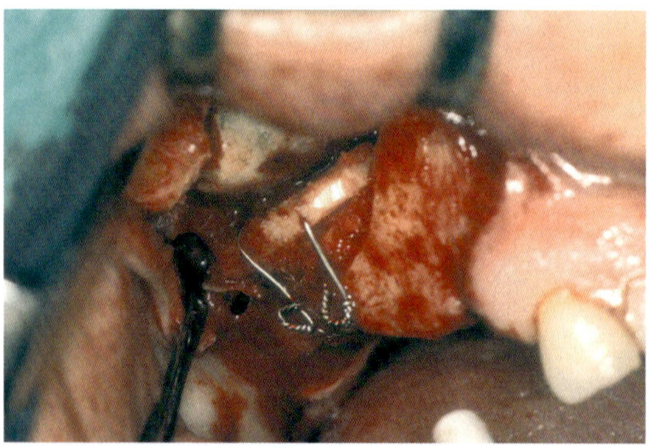

**Figure 5.57** Osteosutures are tightened to keep the bone graft in place.

## 5.3 Impaction of alveolar bone into the maxillary sinus

Methods have been developed to compact alveolar bone into the maxillary sinus by the use of special osteotomy instruments which either impact or infracture bone from the residual alveolar ridge into the sinus cavity. Rosen *et al.* (1999) have reported that by using this technique, between 3–5 mm of bone augmentation can be achieved prior to implant installation. The residual bone volume should be thick enough to allow for impaction to create a residual height of between 8–10 mm. This method is technique-sensitive and there is a risk that the bony floor of sinus will fracture in an unexpected way and cause complications, such as a tear of the sinus membrane.

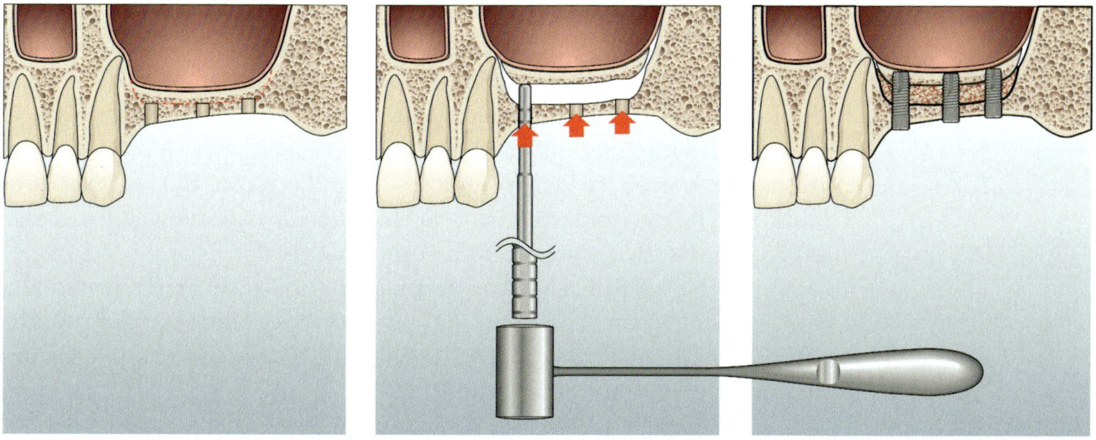

**Figure 5.58** Impaction of alveolar bone with the osteotome technique.

## 5.4 Maxillary osteotomy with interpositional bone graft

Where there has been severe or total atrophy of the alveolar process in the edentulous maxilla it is necessary to graft the entire maxilla thus reconstructing the alveolar process as a whole. Continuous resorption of the alveolar process during long-term denture wear often gives rise to an unfavorable sagittal relationship between the maxillary base and the mandible. In these cases it is not only necessary to reconstruct the bony volume of the alveolar process but also to correct the sagittal relationship between the jaws, facilitating a favorable loading of the implants in an axial direction. The maxillary osteotomy, with the possibility to reposition the maxilla in both the horizontal and vertical direction, is thus the only method to improve the intermaxillary relationship of maxillary base and mandible.

### 5.4.1 *Surgical technique*

A vestibular incision is made with an extension from the first premolar on one side to the corresponding region on the contralateral side. Care should be taken not to extend the incision too far so as not to jeopardize the vascular supply to the maxilla. The nasal apertures and midface region are exposed by reflection of a mucoperiosteal flap. The infraorbital foramina are localized. The nasal mucosa is very gently lifted, taking care not to traumatize or lacerate the tissue. It is inadvisable to have a connection between the nasal cavity and the grafted region in the bony nasal floor. The sinus mucosa in the floor of the sinus recesses is removed before placing the grafts in the cavities.

Bone graft from the iliac crest is modeled to fit into the sinus recesses and nasal floor and cancellous bone is placed underneath. Cortical graft and cancellous bone are mixed together and packed with the cortical part facing superiorly. The grafts are secured with osteosutures and after repositioning of the maxilla in the anterior and inferior directions, the maxilla is fixed with microplates to the midface. One plate is secured on either side of the nasal aperture and, if necessary, cortical grafts are placed in the osteotomy gap between the maxilla and midface. The vestibular incision is closed with continous sutures and left to heal for two weeks before suture removal.

In the case of full maxillary reconstruction, graft material is taken from the iliac crest. The bone graft is allowed to heal for 4–5 months before implant insertion. As with most graft procedures, antibiotics are required during the initial healing phase.

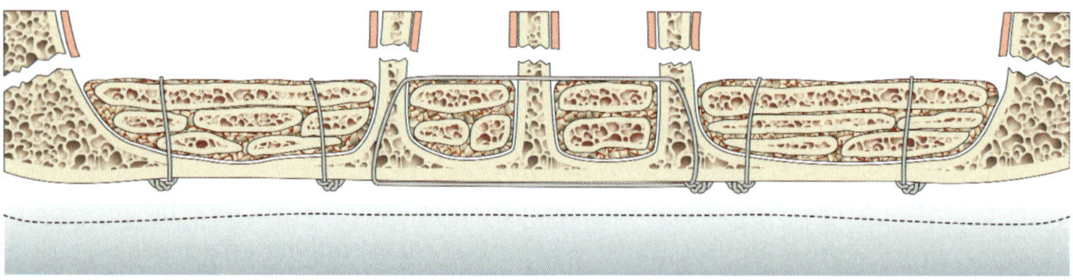

**Figure 5.59** Maxillary osteotomy.

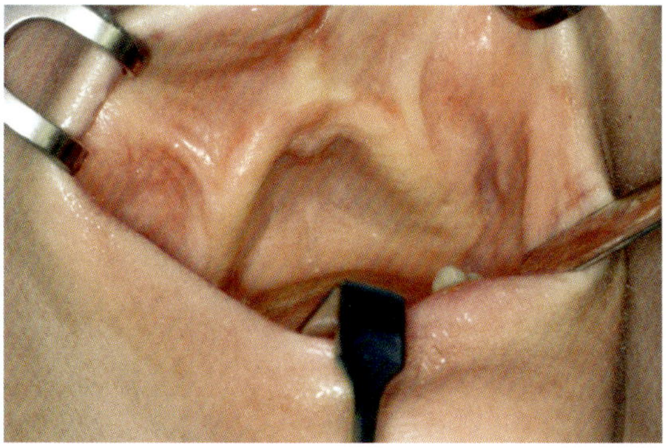

**Figure 5.60** Extreme atrophy of the maxilla.

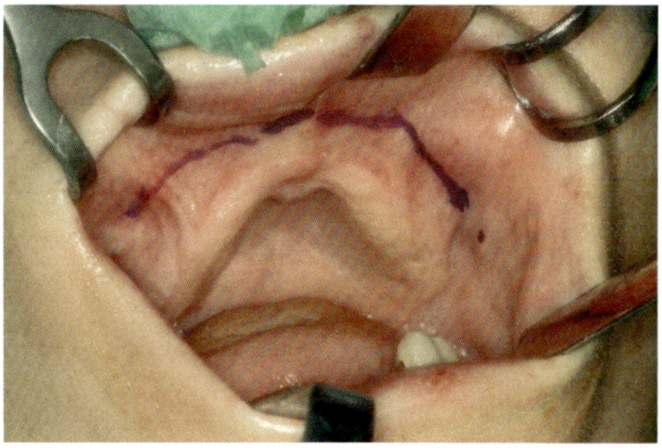

**Figure 5.61** Vestibular incision marked.

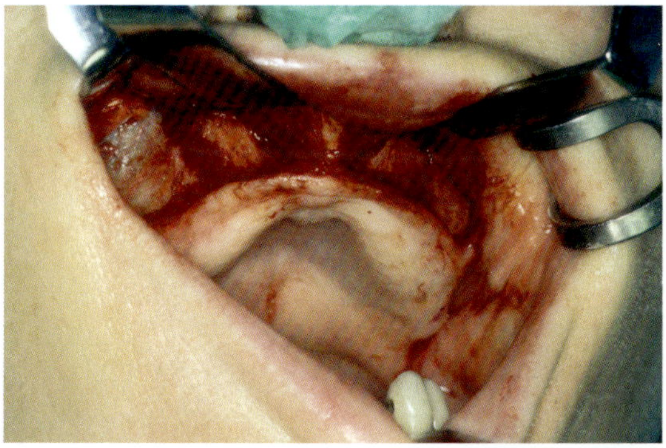

**Figure 5.62** Mucoperiosteal flap elevated and the bony nasal aperture exposed. Note the nasal floor at the level of the crest.

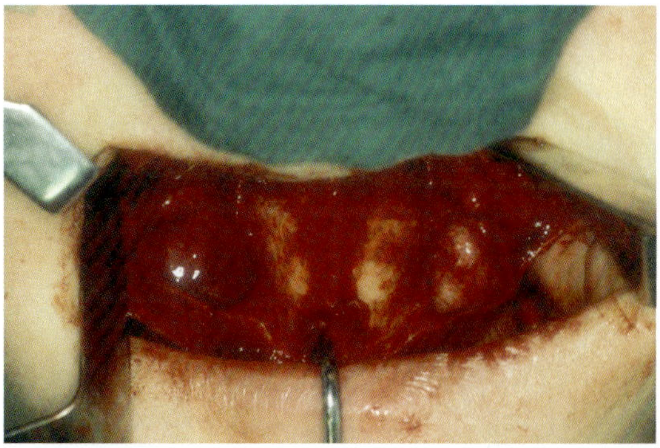

**Figure 5.63** Down-fracture of the resorbed thin maxilla. Sinus cavities and the nasal floor are exposed.

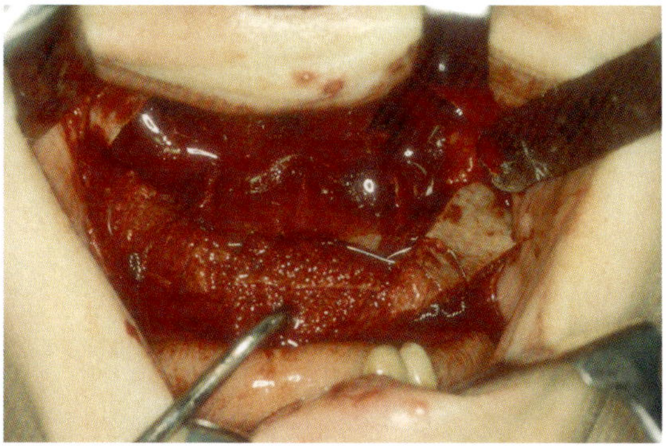

**Figure 5.64** Bone graft from iliac crest is positioned in sinus cavities and nasal floor and is secured with osteosutures.

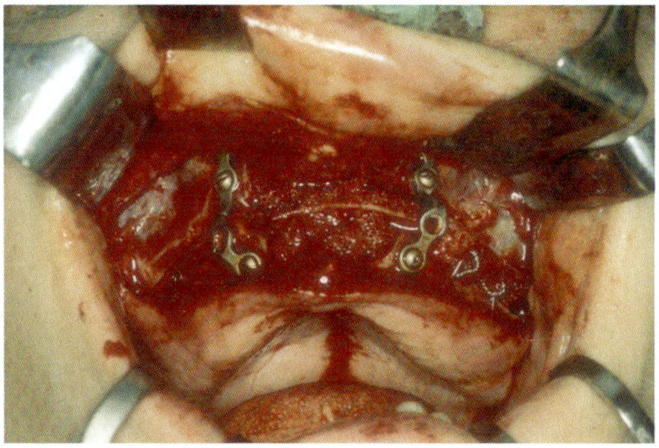

**Figure 5.65** The maxilla is anteriorly and inferiorly repositioned and immobilized with two plates, one on each side of the nasal aperture.

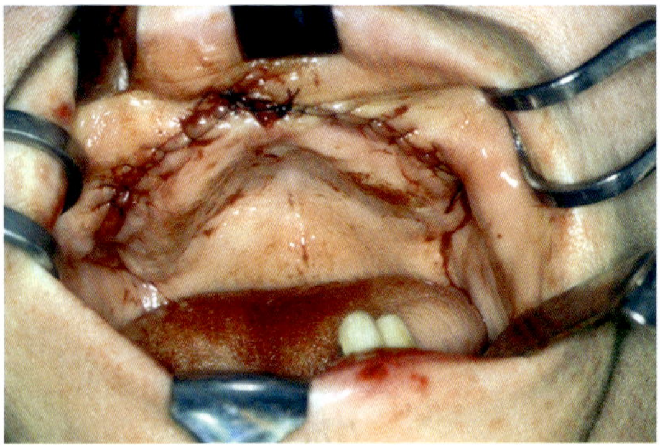

**Figure 5.66** Continuous sutures for closure of vestibular incision.

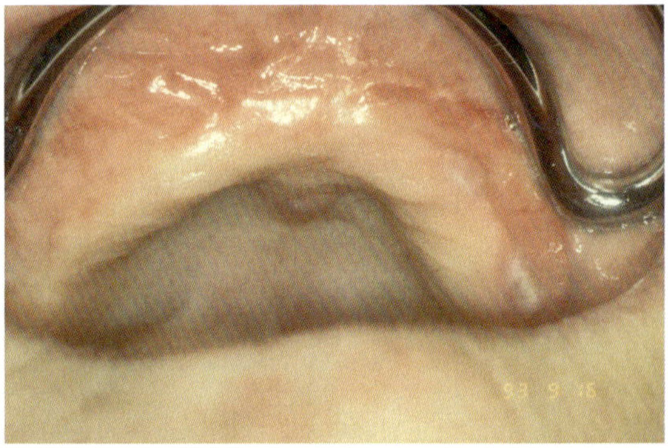

**Figure 5.67** Healing of soft tissues after two weeks.

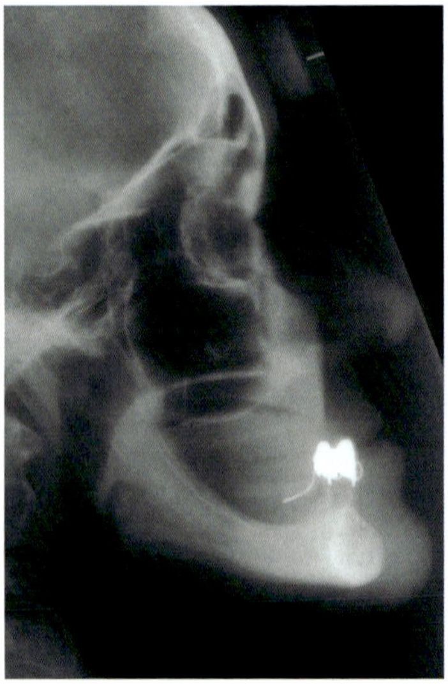

**Figure 5.68** Lateral radiograph preoperatively.

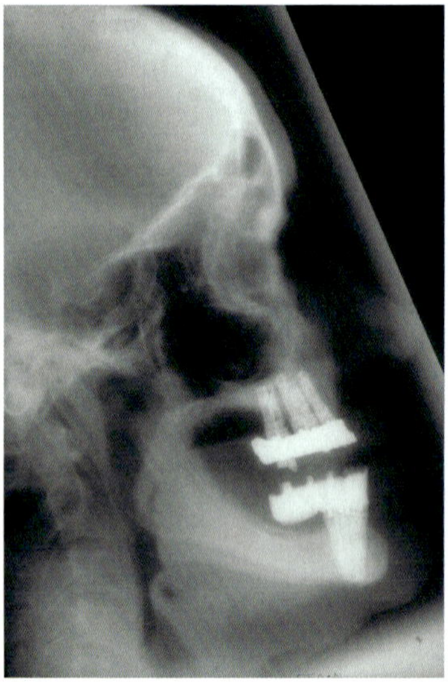

**Figure 5.69** Lateral radiograph after bone grafting and anterior repositioning.

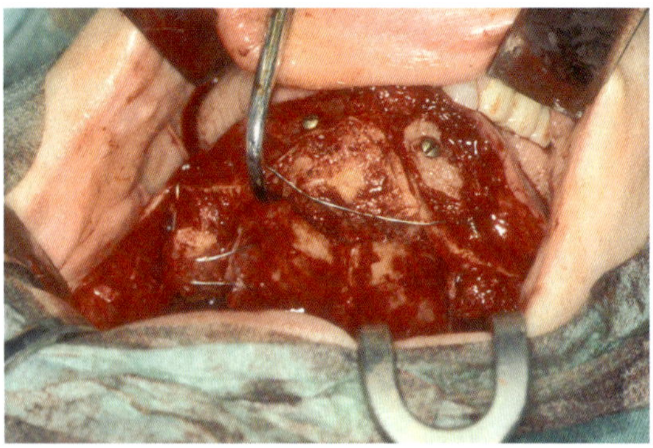

**Figure 5.70** Bone graft and osteosutures in the down-fractured maxilla.

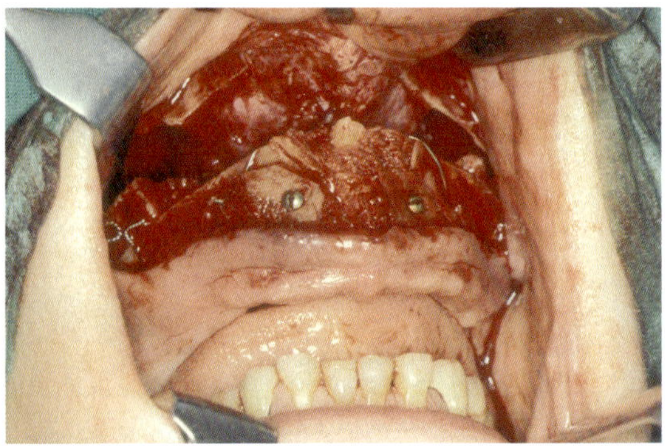

**Figure 5.71** The grafted maxilla is secured with plates on both side of the nasal cavity.

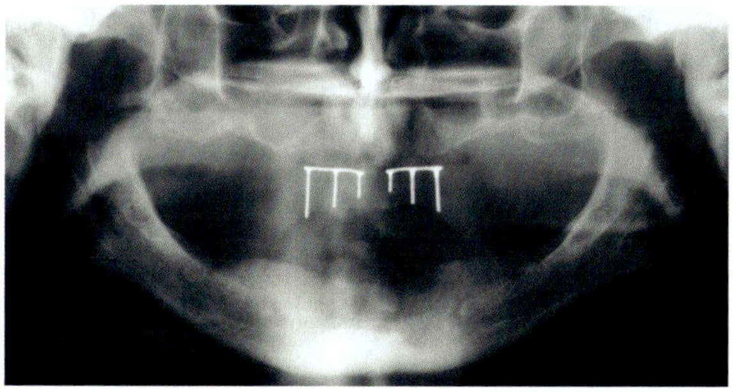

**Figure 5.72** Panoramic radiograph showing an extremely resorbed upper jaw.

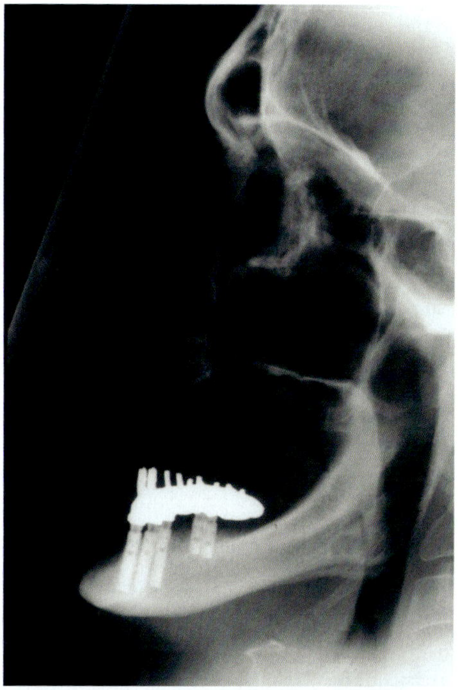

**Figure 5.73** (*right*) Lateral view further illustrates the lack of bone in the maxilla and the retrognathic position.

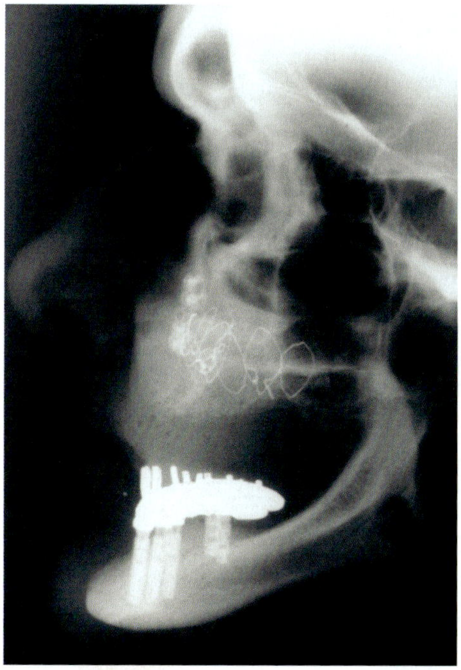

**Figure 5.74** Lateral radiograph after maxillary osteotomy Le Fort I with interpositional bone graft and anterior repositioning of the maxilla.

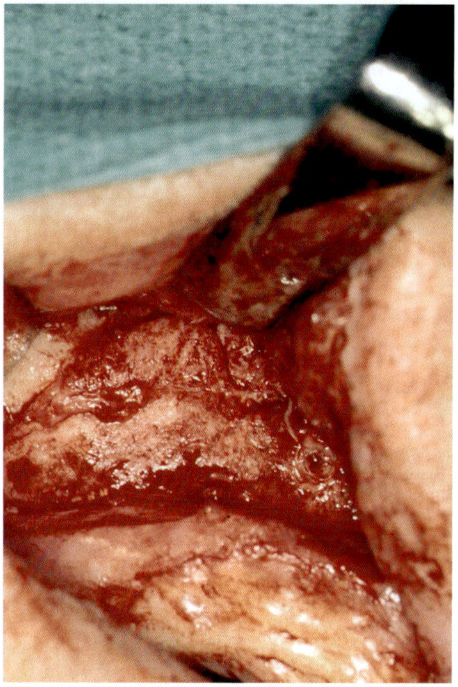

**Figure 5.75** Clinical picture of bone graft healing after 4–5 months.

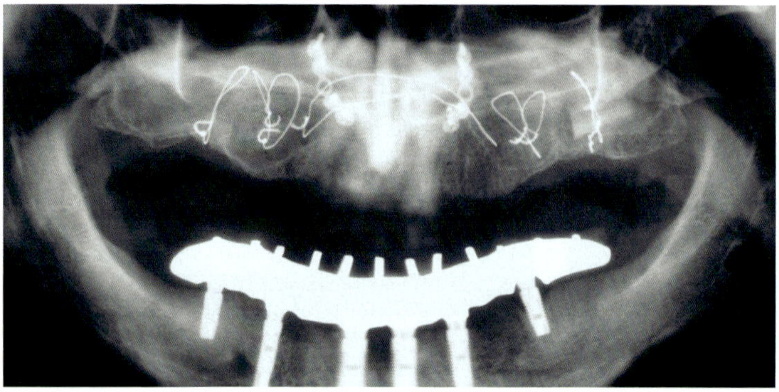

**Figure 5.76** Panoramic radiograph after grafting procedure.

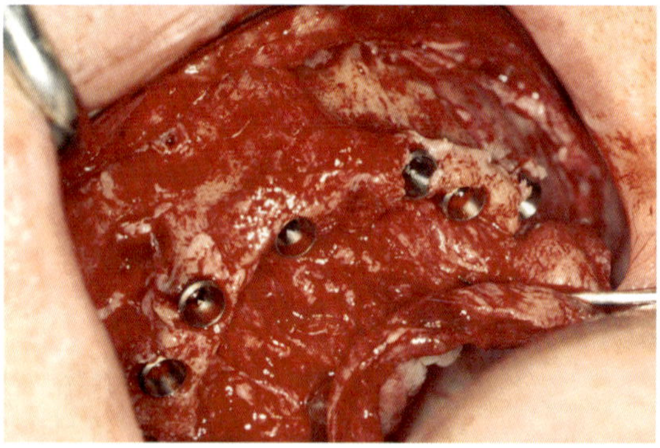

**Figure 5.77** Implants inserted in the grafted maxilla.

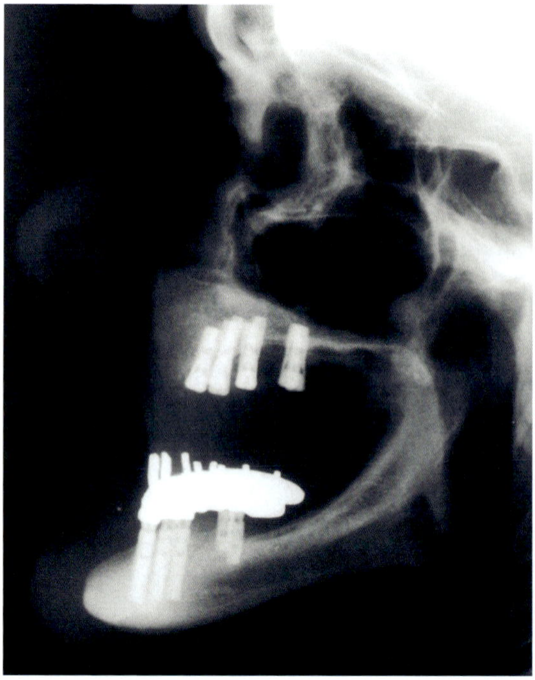

**Figure 5.78** (*right*) Lateral radiograph of the anteriorly repositioned maxilla with implants.

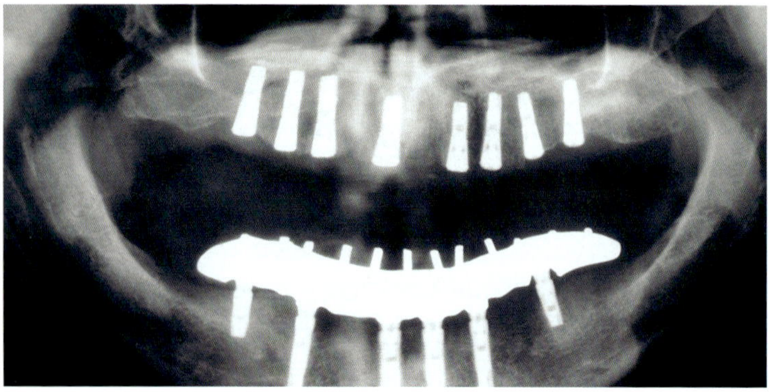

**Figure 5.79** Panoramic view with implants in place.

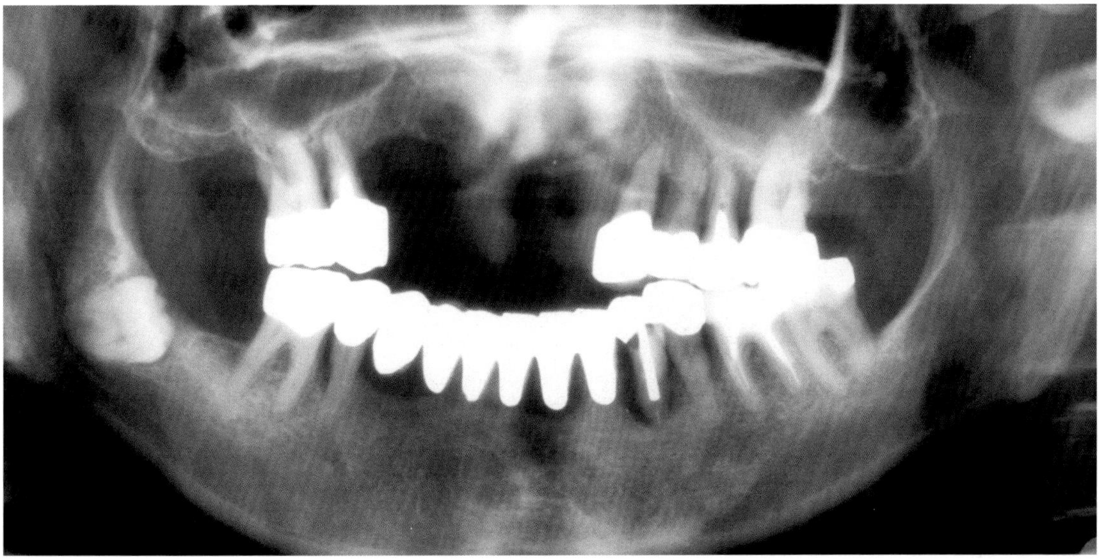

**Figure 5.80** Panoramic radiograph of patient with advanced periodontal and cariogenic disease in his residual dentition of the upper jaw. Note the traumatic loss of the anterior teeth.

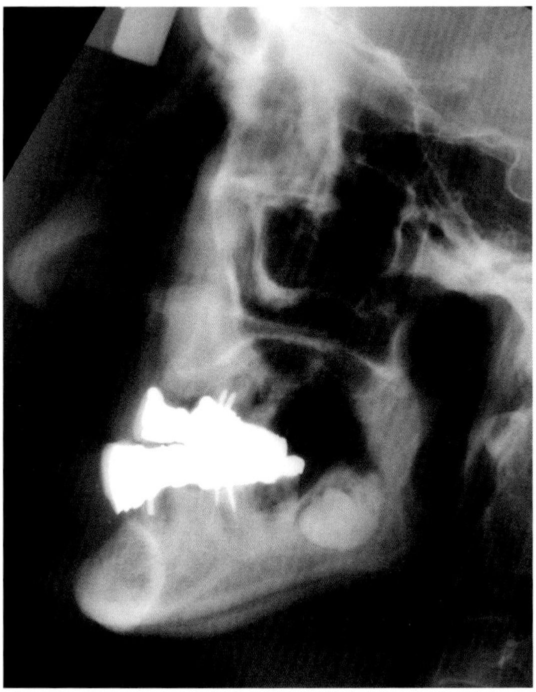

**Figure 5.81** Lateral radiograph showing a retrognathic position of the upper jaw partly due to the traumatic injury.

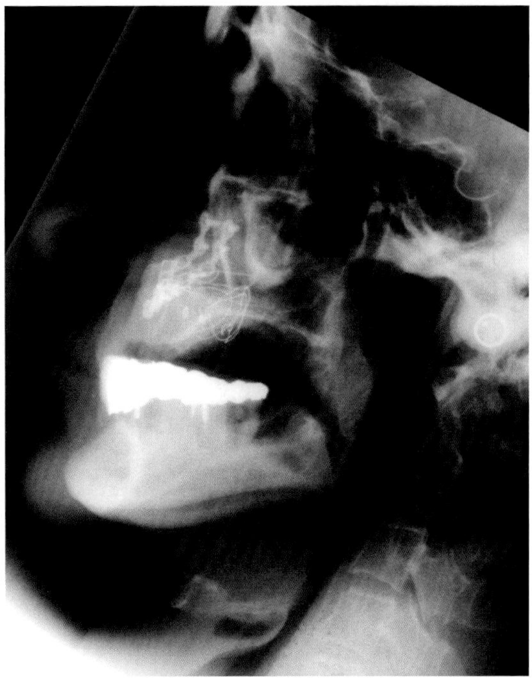

**Figure 5.82** The situation after maxillary osteotomy with anterior repositioning of the maxilla and interpositional bone graft.

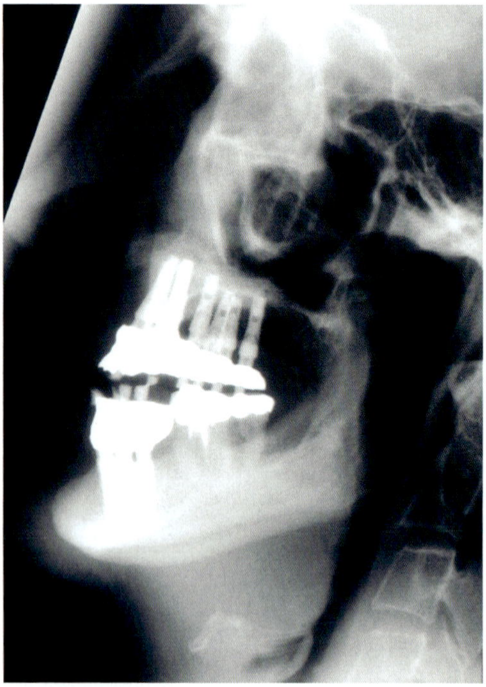

**Figure 5.83** Rehabilitation with implants and bridge.

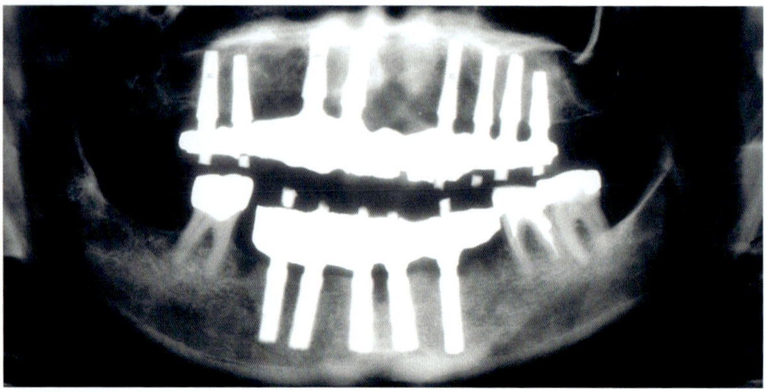

**Figure 5.84** Panoramic radiograph after implant rehabilitation.

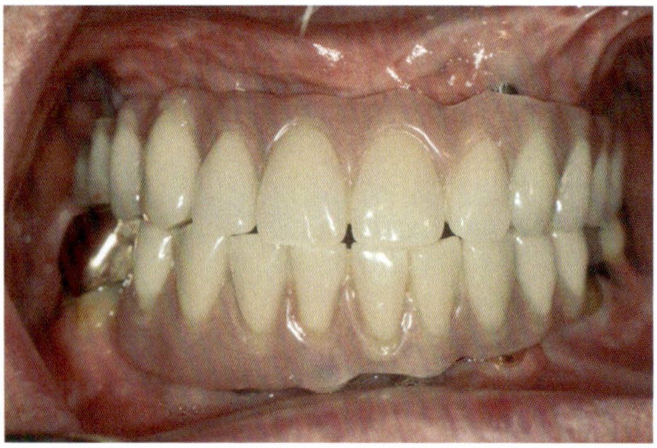

**Figure 5.85** Clinical situation after prosthetic rehabilitation.

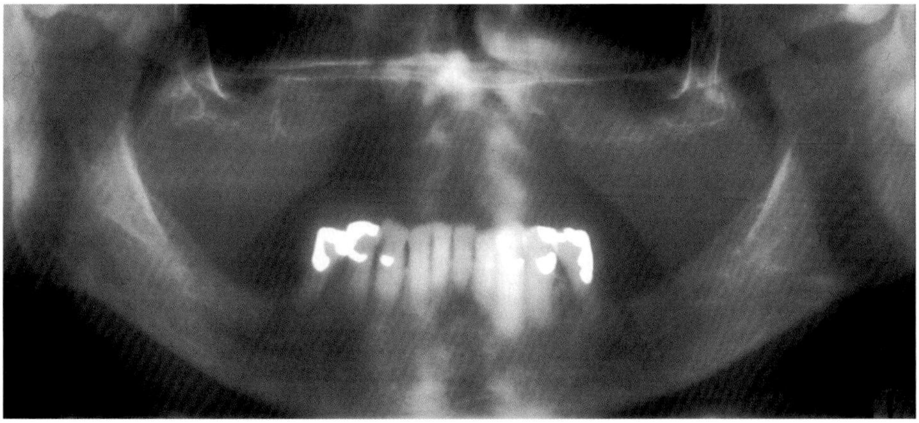

**Figure 5.86** The case illustrates an almost total absence of bone in the maxilla. Lateral radiograph shows very retropositioned maxilla.

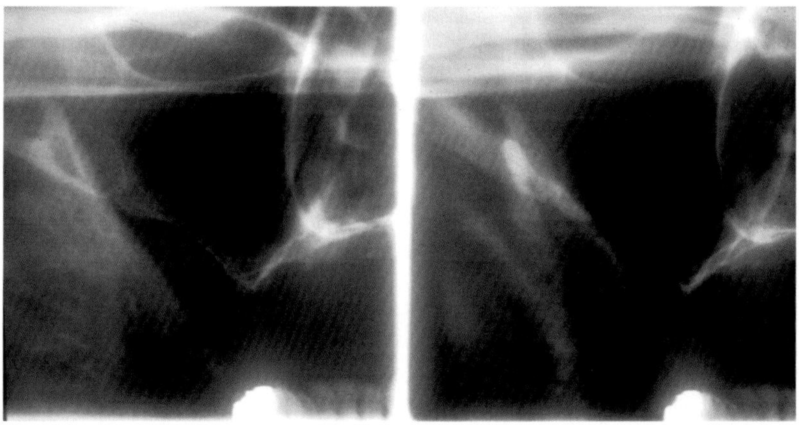

**Figure 5.87a** Scanora tomography showing absence of bone beneath the sinus cavity.

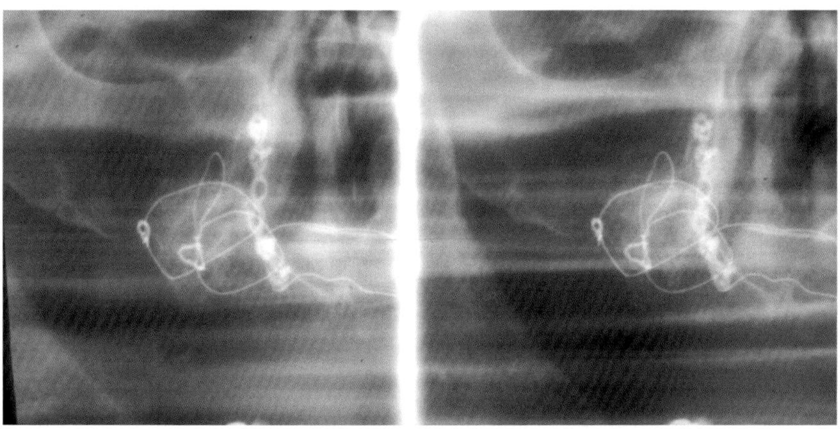

**Figure 5.87b** The same projection with bone graft in place.

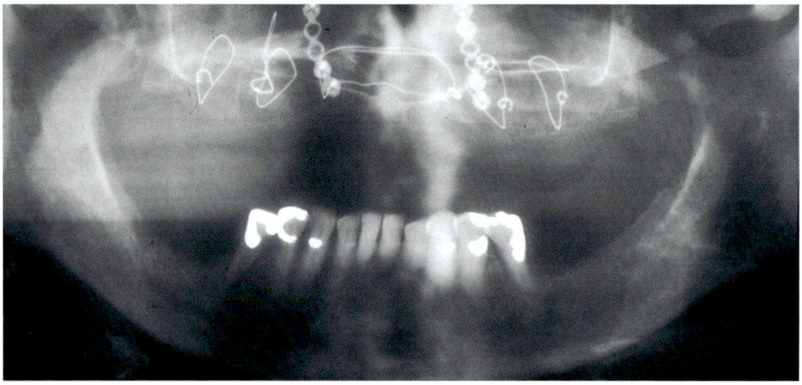

**Figure 5.88** Panoramic view after bone grafting.

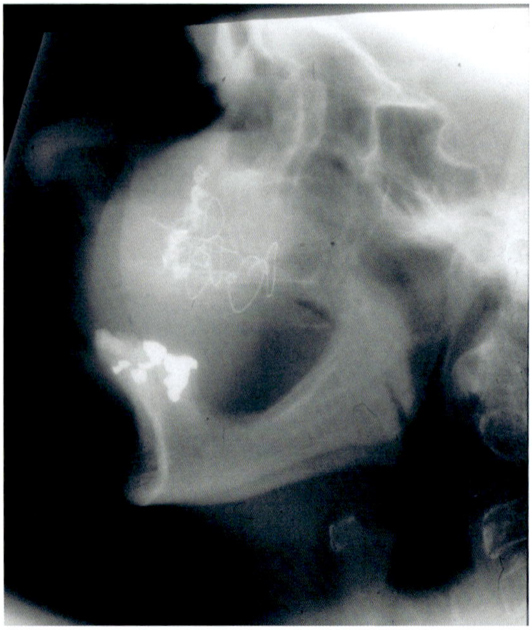

**Figure 5.89** Lateral radiograph after bone grafting showing a better sagittal relation.

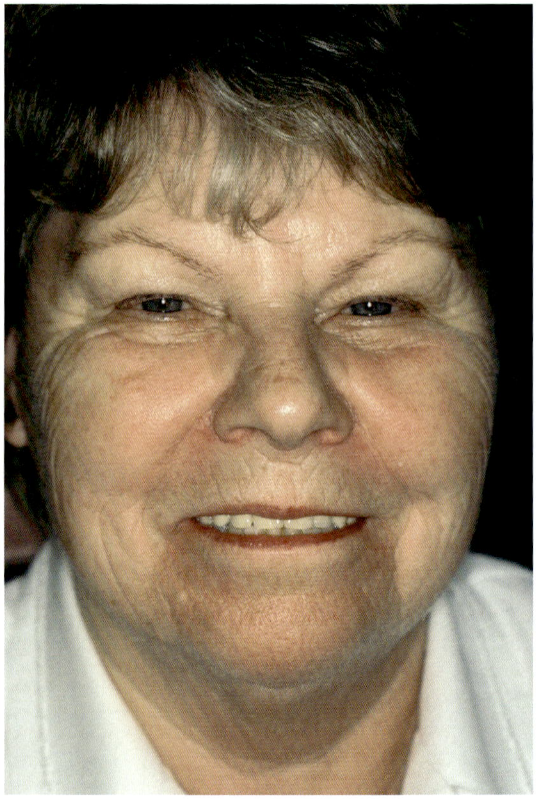

**Figure 5.90** The patient after prosthetic rehabilitation.

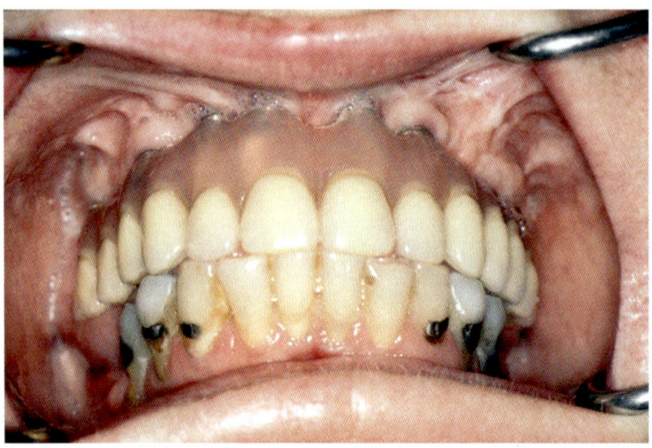

**Figure 5.91** Clinical view of bridge reconstruction.

# 6 Segmental Osteotomy for Bone Augmentation Procedures

## 6.1 Indication

This procedure can be used for patients with a low height of the alveolar process but a satisfactory width. It is also suitable for localized defects of the alveolar process such as those caused by trauma defects.

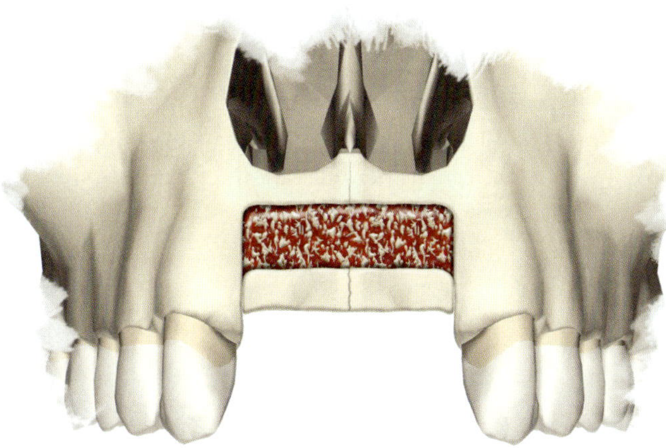

**Figure 6.1** Segmental osteotomy.

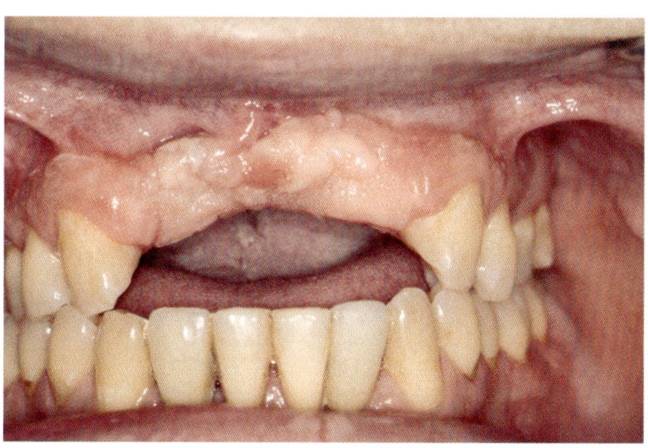

**Figure 6.2** Traumatic injury with loss of teeth and alveolar bone in the maxillary anterior region.

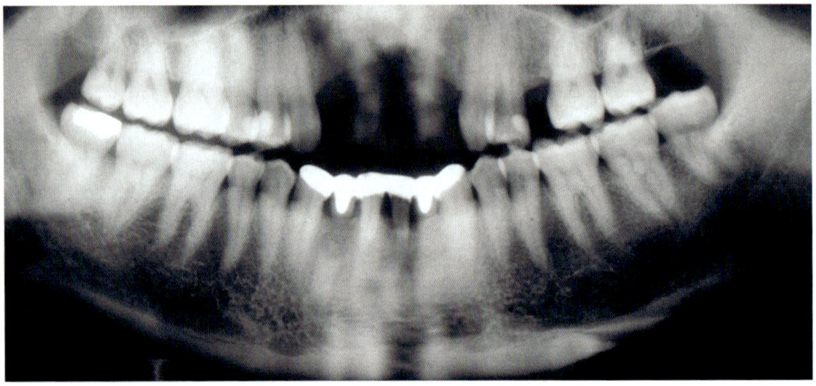

**Figure 6.3** Panoramic view of the situation.

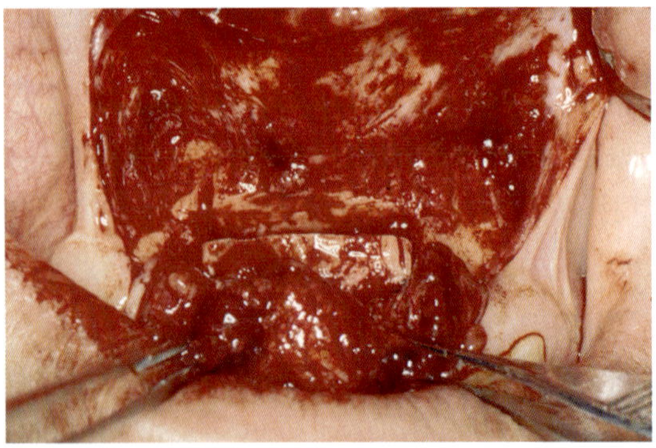

**Figure 6.4** Vestibular incision with exposure of the alveolar process and segmental osteotomy of the edentulous portion.

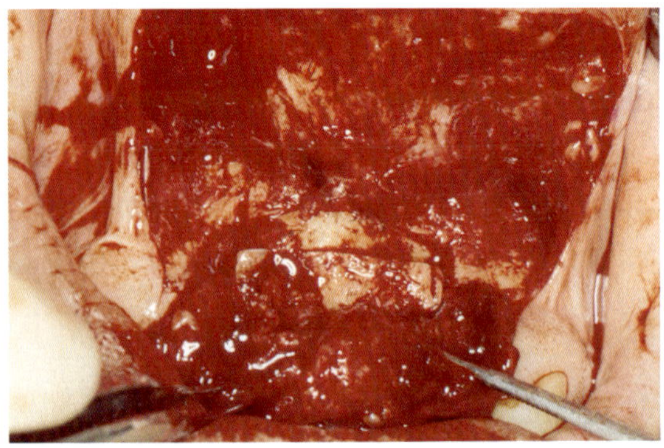

**Figure 6.5** Bone graft from the chin is positioned in the gap after elevation of the segment to increase the alveolar height.

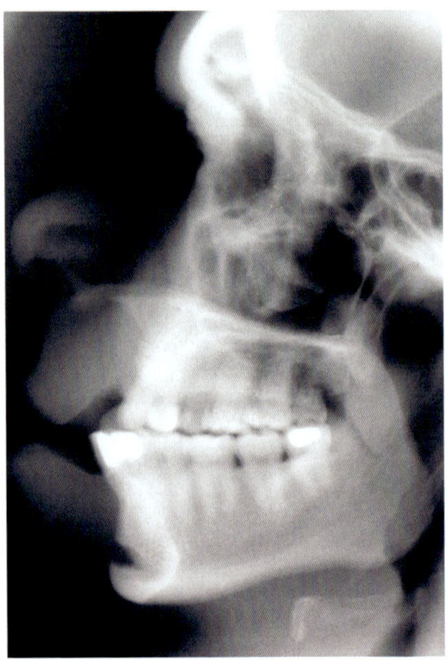

**Figure 6.6** Lateral radiograph visualizing the bone graft site.

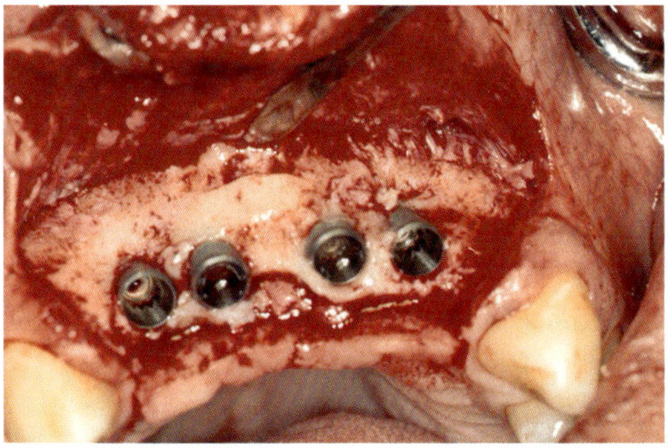

Figure 6.7 Implants inserted in elevated segment.

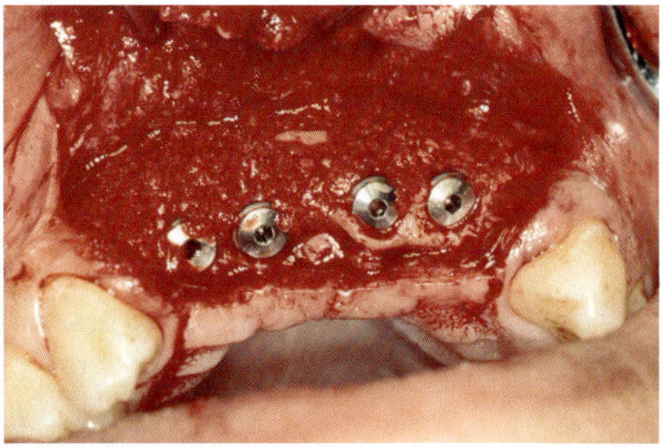

Figure 6.8 Bone material from BoneTrap™ smoothing the bone surface.

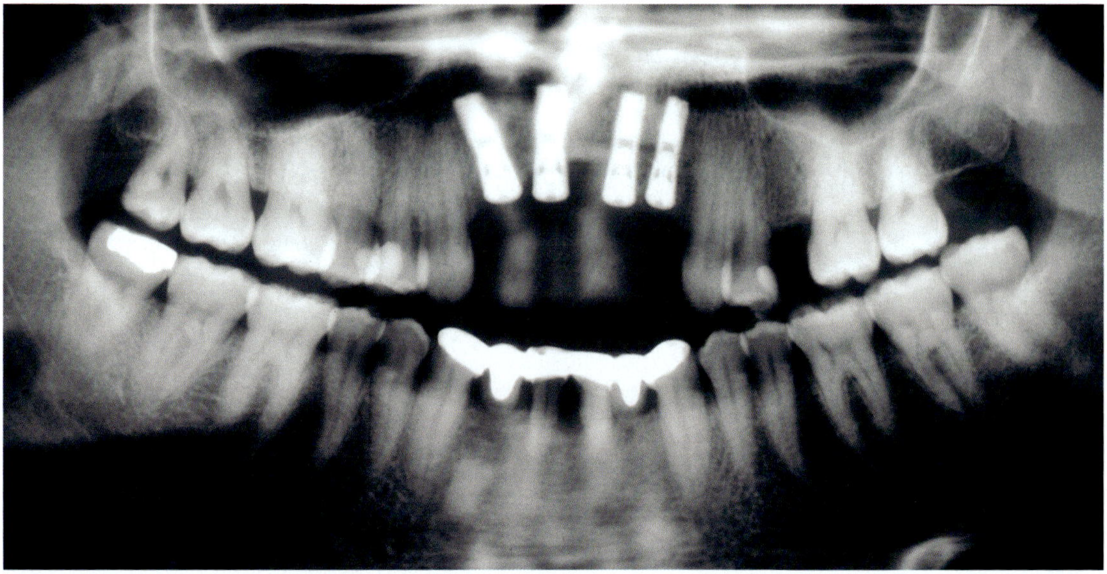

Figure 6.9 Panoramic radiograph of implants in place.

## 6.2 Surgical technique

The primary objective is to maintain the vitality of the segment. Incisions should be made in the vestibular sulcus maintaining the vascular supply from the lateral mucosa and from the lingual and palatal mucosa, respectively.

Using an oscillating saw with a thin blade, an osteotomy is made horizontally a couple of millimetres from the crest and joined with two vertical cuts, all of them through the bone tissue but not perforating the periosteum and the mucosa. The segment is mobilized within the elastic limits of the soft tissues and a cortical bone graft of the desired thickness sandwiched between the base of the alveolar process and the segment. Bone plates are used to immobilize both the segment and the graft material.

Mobilization of the segment is easier in the mandible due to the elasticity of the mucosal tissue whereas in the maxilla the firm adhesion of the palatal mucosa makes the mobility more difficult. In the maxilla there is a tendency for palatal tilting of the segment. Careful suturing is advocated to prevent communication to the oral cavity. Healing takes 4–6 months, depending on the cortical character of the bone graft.

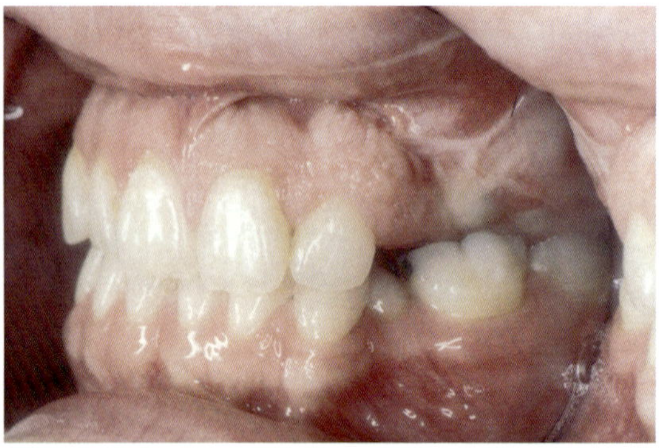

**Figure 6.10** A patient with fibrous dysplasia where the posterior edentulous maxilla had increased in height preventing occlusal rehabilitation.

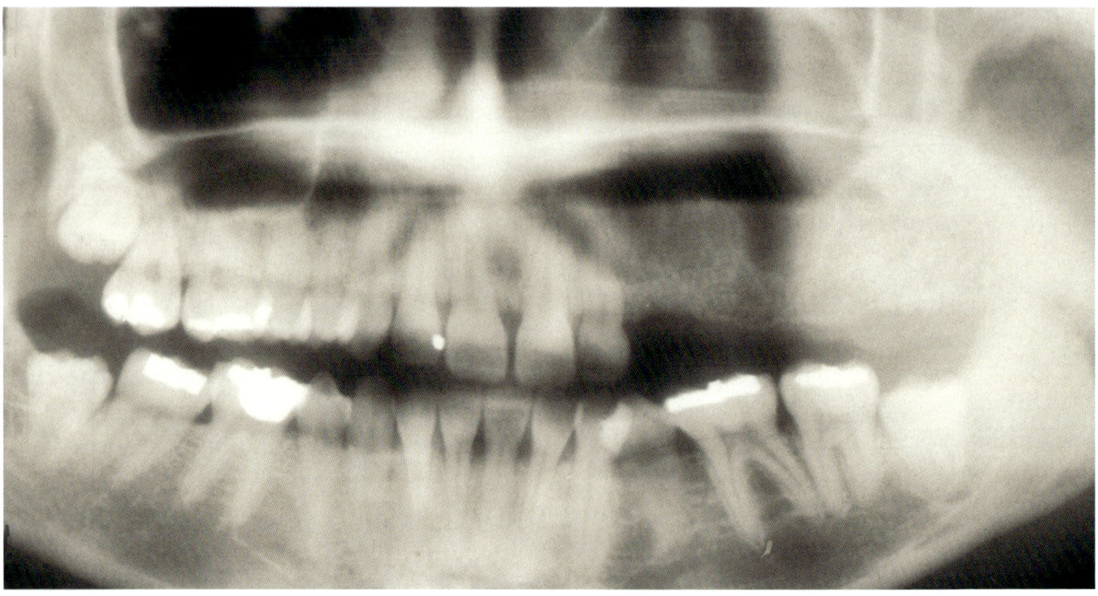

**Figure 6.11** The clinical situation with no space between dentition in the lower jaw and the opposing alveolar crest.

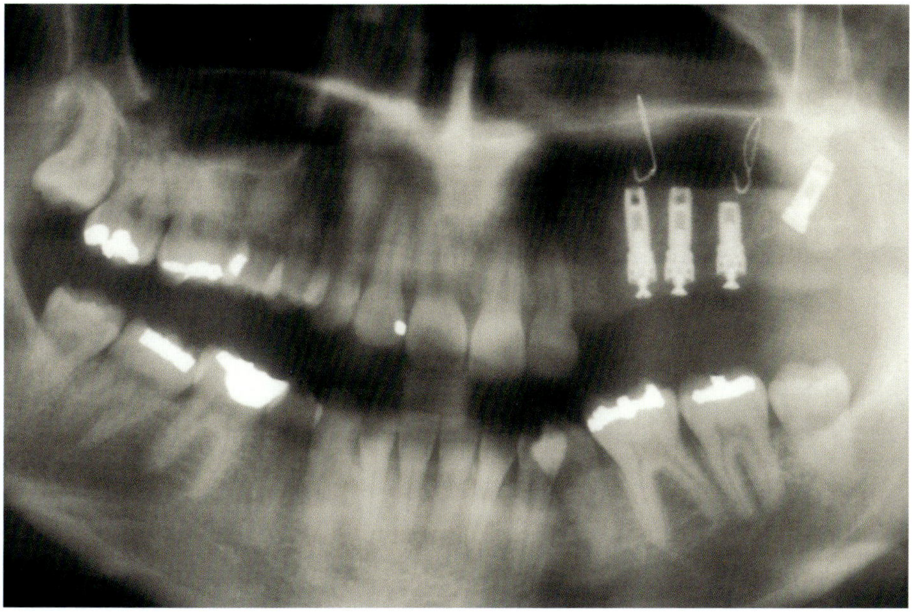

**Figure 6.12** Surgical intrusion of segment and insertion of implants.

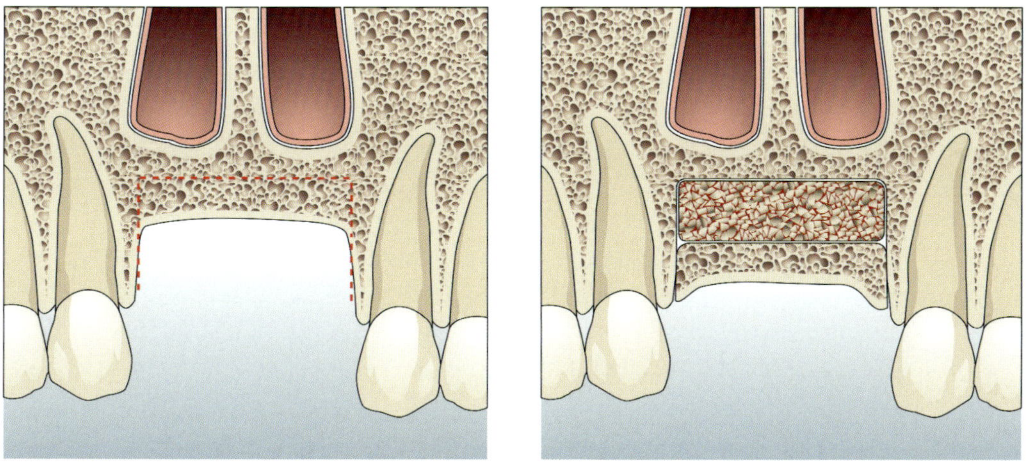

**Figure 6.13** Segmental osteotomy with bone graft.

# 7 Distraction Osteogenesis for the Augmentation Of The Alveolar Process

## 7.1 Indication

This is suitable for localized defects of the alveolar process with a reduced height but a wide alveolar base.

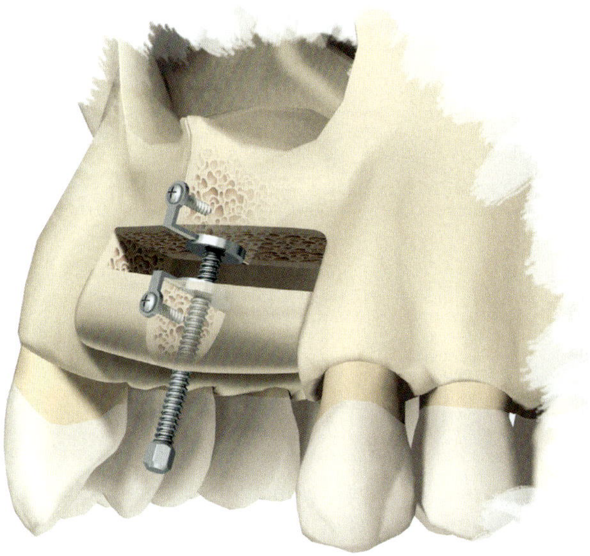

**Figure 7.1** Distraction.

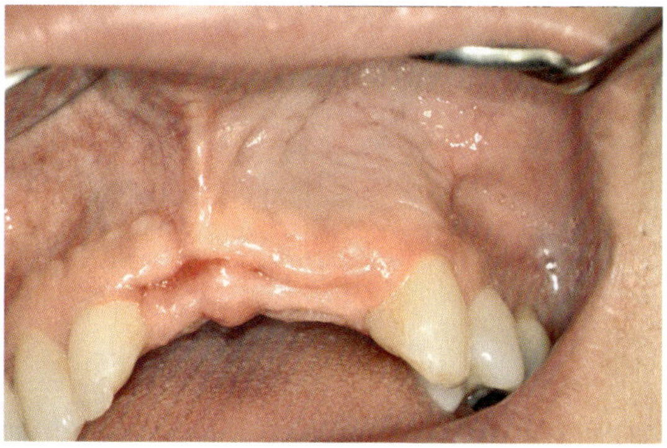

**Figure 7.2** Clinical situation in a patient after traumatic loss of teeth and bone.

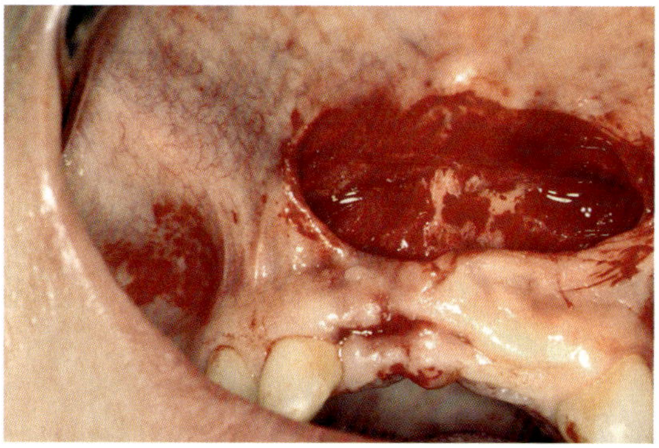

**Figure 7.3** Vestibular incision and exposure of the alveolar process.

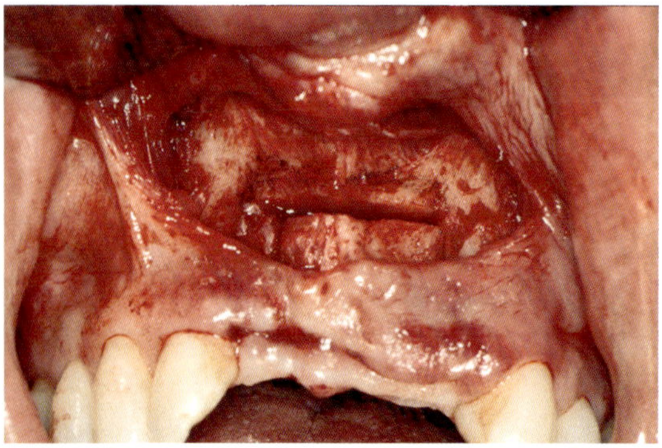

**Figure 7.4** Segmental osteotomy performed with a thin oscillating saw blade.

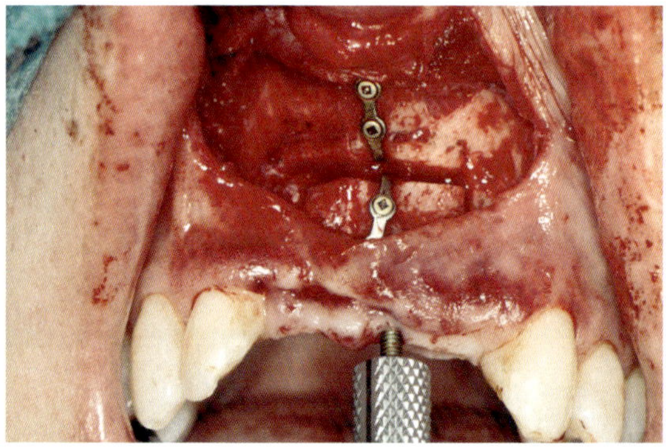

**Figure 7.5** Thin plates (stop plate and distraction plate) are secured in the bone segment and the alveolar base. The distraction screw is introduced through the segment.

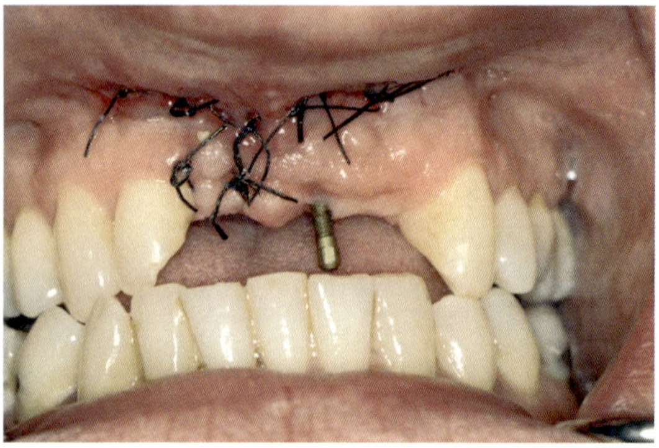

**Figure 7.6** Clinical view after healing period.

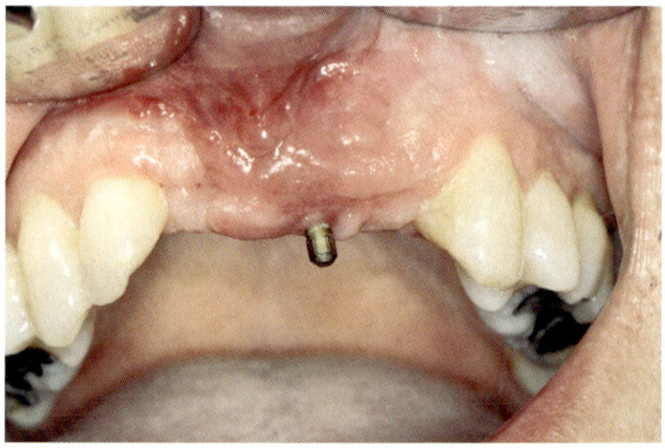

**Figure 7.7** After distraction for one week the segment is elevated.

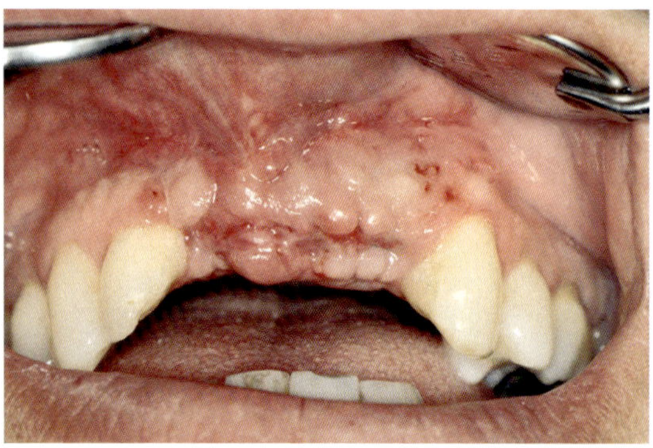

**Figure 7.8** The final situation with distracted segment.

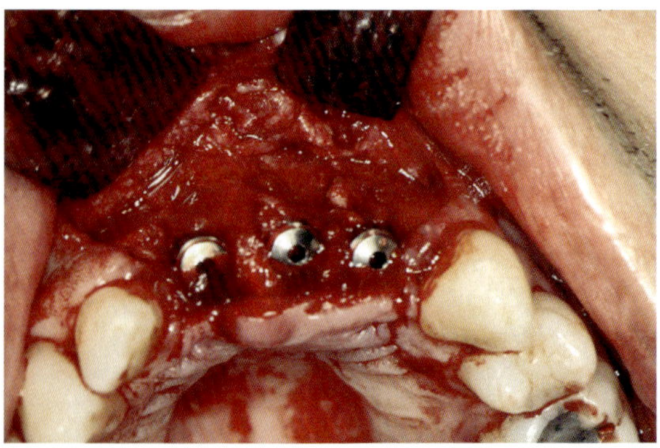

**Figure 7.9** Insertion of implants.

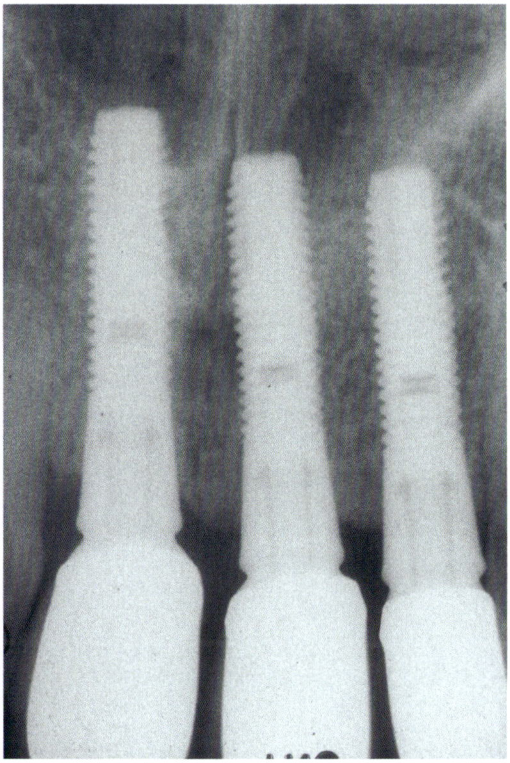

Figure 7.10 Radiograph showing implants in place.

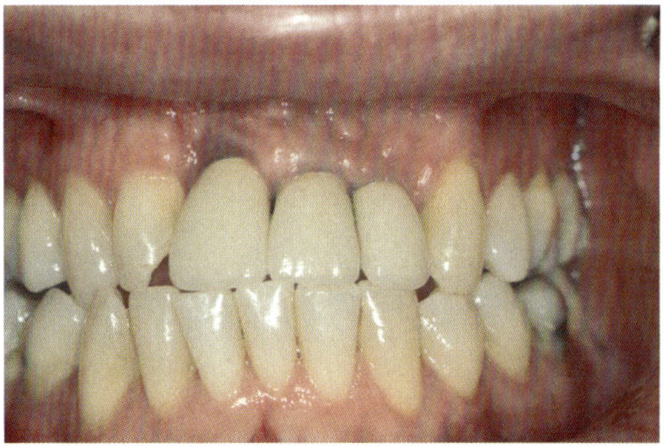

Figure 7.11 Rehabilitation with a bridge.

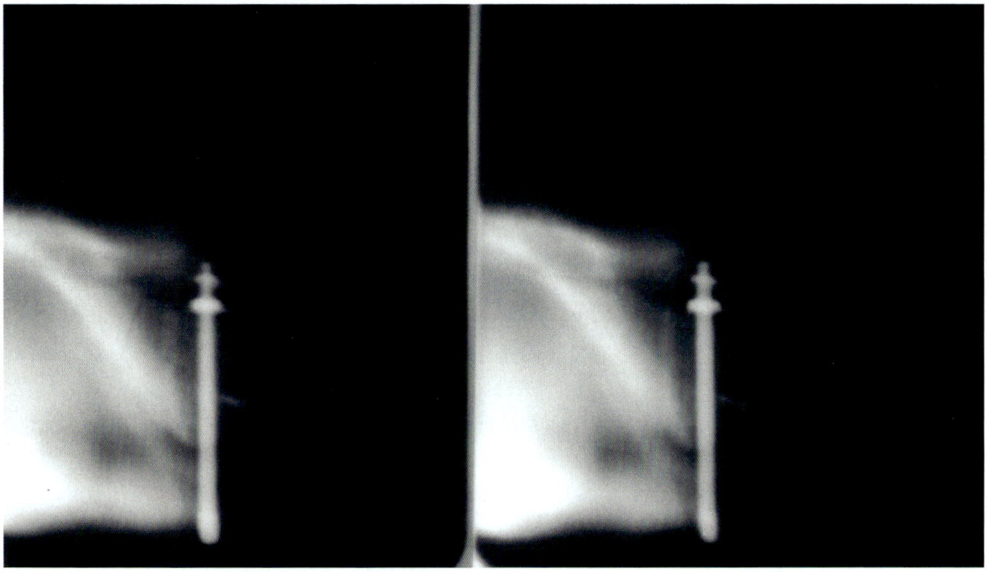

Figure 7.12 Tomography before the start of distraction.

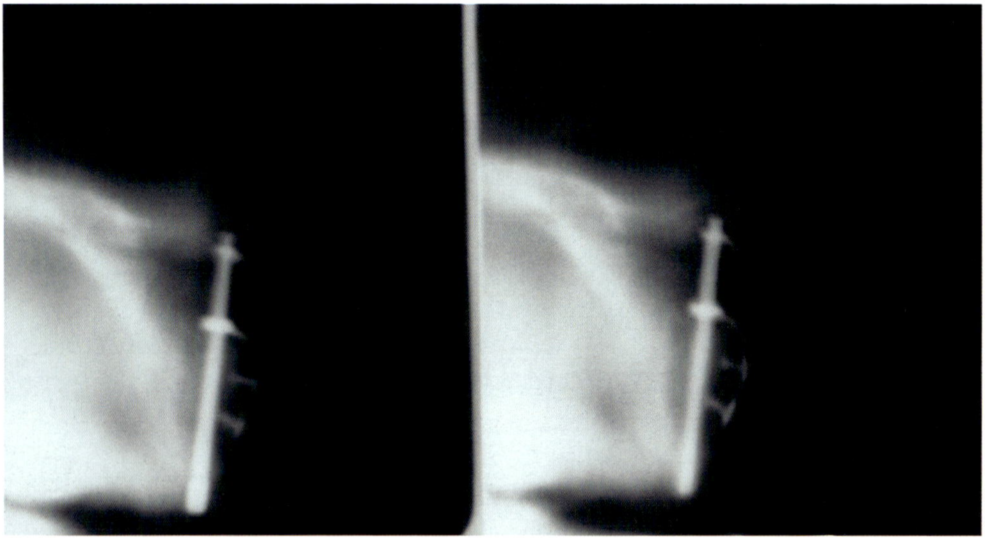

**Figure 7.13** Tomography showing 7–8 mm distraction osteogenesis.

## 7.2 Surgical technique

Distraction allows for continuous bone formation while the bone surfaces are slowly separated. Vestibular incision is mandatory to maintain the vascular supply to the segment that will be distracted. An intact periosteum is an important prerequisite for successful bone regeneration.

An osteotomy cut is made through the cortical plates and also through the intermediate cancellous bone. The segment to be distracted is mobilized and distraction devices introduced. These devices are generally composed of two titantium plates, one of which is fixed to the mobilized segment and the other to the alveolar base. The distraction screw penetrates the segment plate and is tapered to fit through the segment plate hole. The base plate has a stop hole for the screw, enabling the segment to be distracted away from the bone base. The incision is then closed by careful suturing and left to heal for a couple of weeks.

After primary soft tissue healing, the distraction screw is turned through 0.4 mm each day for ten days, thus achieving 4 mm distraction of the segment. Depending on the anatomical situation, further distraction can of course be undertaken.

After completing the distraction phase, consolidation of the distraction area proceeds for 6–8 weeks. After the distraction device is removed, implant surgery is then carried out in the conventional manner.

Distraction osteogenesis can be carried out in any part of the alveolar process provided that there is enough bone to segmentalize without intruding into the nerve canal or maxillary sinus. Distraction osteogeneis has the same indication as segmental osteotomy but the gradual distraction of tissues makes it more suitable in difficult situations where it is more or less impossible to mobilize a segment. The palatal mucosa in the upper jaw is such an example where segmentation often results in tilting of the segment palatally.

A problem with the distraction method is of course that it does not change the form of the alveolar process, so if there is a defect such as an unfavorable contour this will persist after distraction. However, distraction osteogenesis has its place in augmentation procedures in both the maxilla and mandible as a complement to other bone regeneration methods.

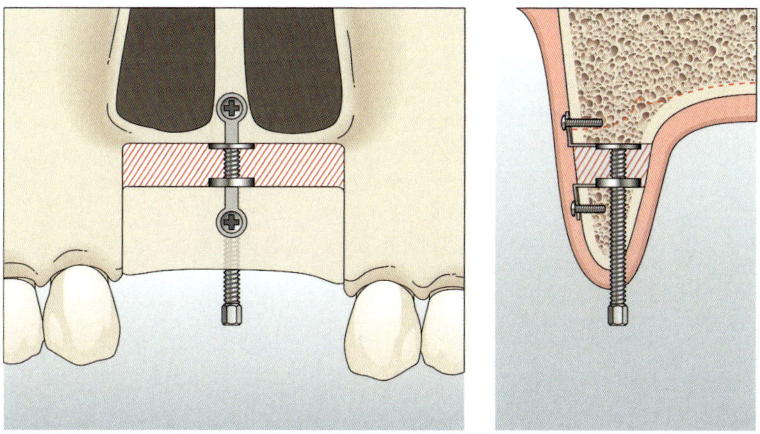

**Figure 7.14** Distraction technique.

# 8 Complications

## 8.1 Grafting sites

With grafting procedures, as with all surgical operations, there is a risk of complications. These may be associated with the grafting methods, healing of the grafts and, of course, with implant integration in the graft material. In severe cases, iliac crest bone grafting can result in perforations to the abdominal cavity, hernia formation, defective ridge healing or fracture of the crest, in addition to the more frequent post-operative problems such as pain and limited movement of the affected leg for some time.

Grafting from the tibia may give rise to pain for a limited time and in cases where undermining of the bone has been too severe there is also a risk of fracture.

Mandibular bone grafts from the mental region can initiate severe bleeding into the floor of the mouth especially in the case of bicortical grafts. Such a complication can be fatal in the worst cases, due to airway obstruction. When the osteotomy is performed too close to the apices of the lower teeth, devitalisation and sensitivity disturbances can occur. Neuralgia problems from interference with the anterior branch of the inferior alveolar nerve is another problematic complication. Pain often occurs from this region after grafting.

Grafts from the mandibular angle and ramus region typically result in less pain but almost always cause considerable swelling. There is a risk of traumatizing the inferior alveolar nerve if the split is made too medial in the mandibular body. Grafting from the alveolar process is dependent on the extent of the graft and its relationship to adjoining anatomical structures.

With calvarial bone grafts it is technically possible to interfere with the intracranial structures if the grafting technique breaches the inner cortical table.

## 8.2 Onlay grafting

With onlay grafting, complications that may arise are graft exposure due to insufficient mucosal coverage, tension breakdown of the flap or insufficient vascular supply to the mucoperiosteum. In these cases all, or part, of the bone graft will be resorbed and eventually will have to be removed. If implants are inserted simultaneously one or several of these will be lost. Resorption of onlay grafts will always be a complication in those parts which are not functionally stimulated. Mobilization of the graft due to trauma from dentures or pressure from chewing may initiate inflammatory processes and consequently bone graft failure.

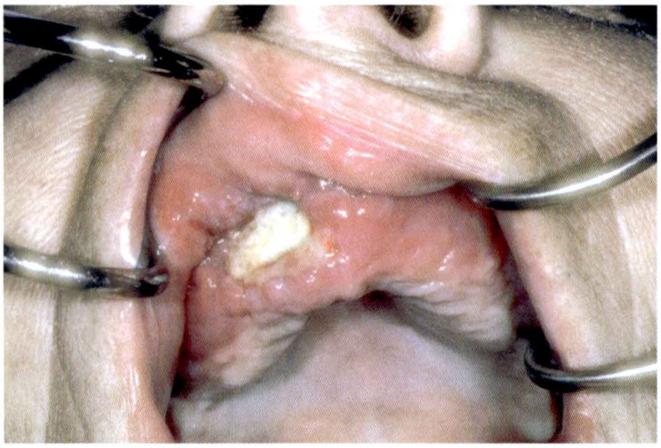

**Figure 8.1** Partial exposure of large onlay graft. Secondary healing with loss of some of the graft material.

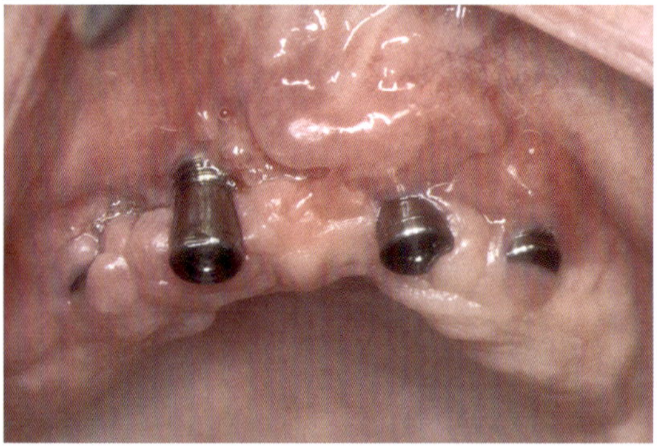

**Figure 8.2** Trauma from dentures with exposure of cover screws and part of the implants.

## 8.3 Inlay grafts

Regarding the maxillary osteotomy procedure, surgical complications may arise such as nerve damage, intra-operative and post-operative bleedings. Severely resorbed maxillae are often so thin that they may easily fracture unless treated very carefully. It is important to keep the nasal mucosa intact to prevent nasal bacteria infecting the graft. If perforations should occur, it is essential that they are repaired by tight suturing. Bone graft fragments which are not stabilized may also give rise to inflammation.

There must be a good bony contact between the grafted maxilla and the bony midface. If the maxilla has a poor bony contact pseudarthroses may occur. This can also happen if the maxilla is loaded too early. However, wound dehiscences, which may occur in onlay grafting, are very seldom seen in the inlay procedure.

Sinus lifting procedures may be associated with complications such as sinusitis and graft loss if the sinus membrane is lacerated or perforated. If blood or foreign particles enter the sinus cavity, the risk of complications is obvious and an infection may be easily established due to the minimal drainage from – and ventilation to – the sinus cavity. Curing an established sinus infection is also difficult and so chronic sinus infections should be taken into account before beginning the procedure. Loosening of graft material may also be an infection risk, and if implants and graft material are inserted simultaneously within a narrow alveolar ridge a micromobility could arise in the whole complex with subsequent loss of both implants and graft along with serious post-operative complications such as an oro-antral fistula formation.

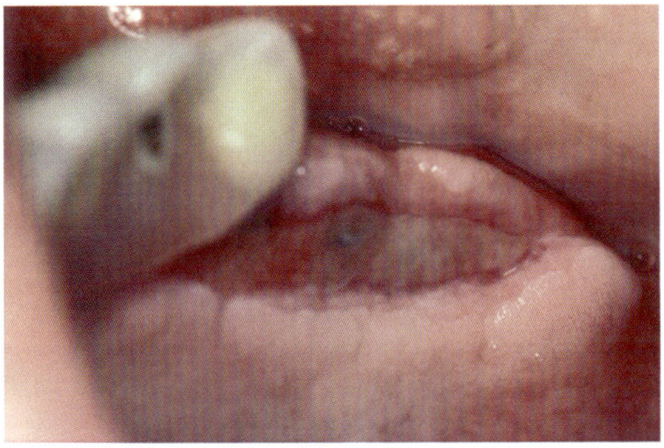

**Figure 8.3** Wound dehiscences after crestal incision in connection with sinus grafting.

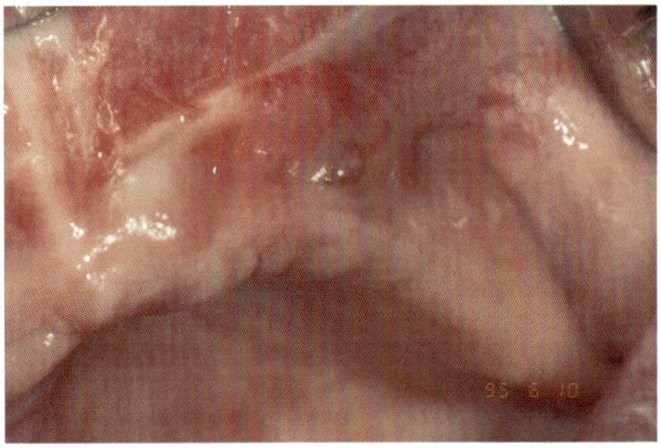

**Figure 8.4** Sinusitis with fistula after sinus lifting procedure.

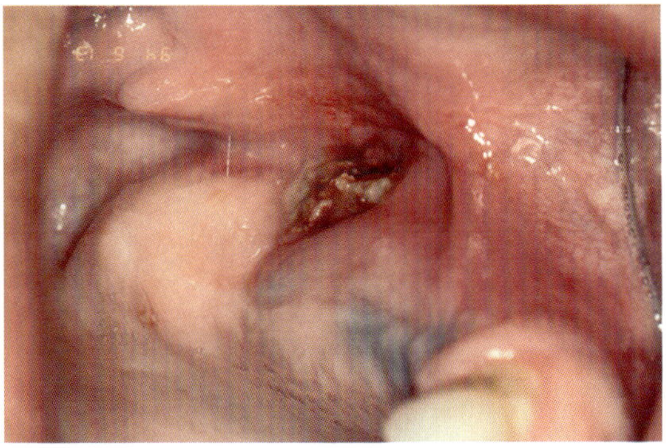

**Figure 8.5** Sequestration of bone graft in maxillary sinus.

# 9 Bone Substitutes in Maxillary Reconstruction Procedures

## 9.1 Bone substitutes

In the search for alternative materials to mix with bone or substitute for bone grafts, a number of different compounds have been tried in the clinical setting. Hydroxyapatite is the major component of normal bone and teeth and has been used in augmentation procedures for many years before the implant era. It has a great affinity for bone tissue and can act as a hard but less vascularized augmentation material. Fibrous tissue may invade between the particles if it is used in a particulized form. The same pattern appears when Bio-Oss®, a choralline substance from bovine bone, is used in the clinical setting. However, mixing the bone substitute material with autologous bone in a 50:50 ratio has more successful results. Hence, the use of these alloplastic and xenograft materials may mean it is possible to reduce the amount of bone graft to be harvested.

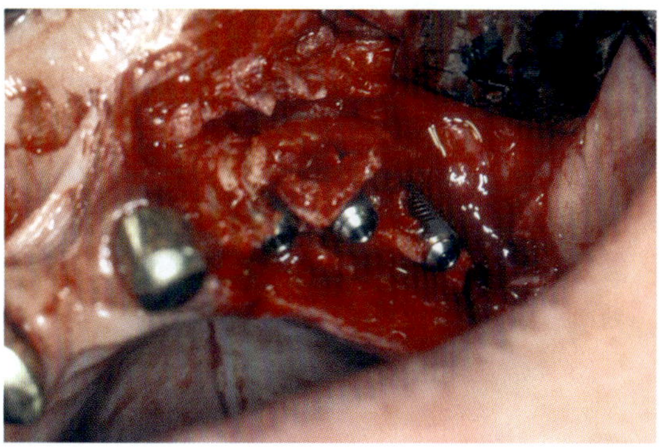

**Figure 9.1** Patient with bone deficiency around inserted implant.

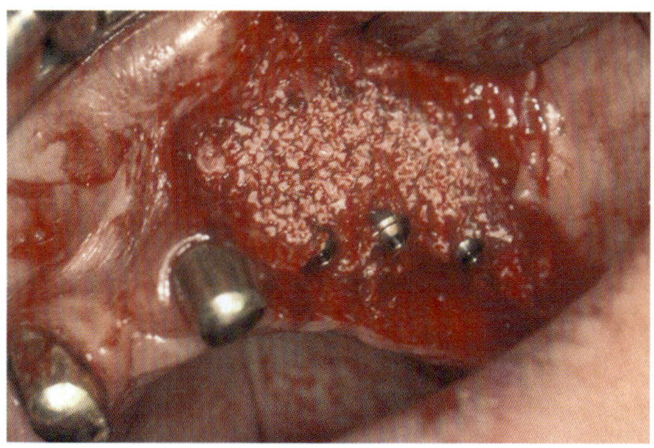

**Figure 9.2** Bio-Oss® granules are used to improve stability and increase width of alveolar crest.

# 10 Summary and Conclusion

At the start of the modern implant era, only patients with adequate bone volume were candidates for implant rehabilitation. The lower jaw was considered the most important area to rehabilitate with implants. With the passage of time, however, the maxilla also became the subject of implant treatment. The bone quality and amount of bone available was often variable and commonly there was a deficiency of bone volume. Brånemark and collaborators (Adell *et al.* 1990b) typically attempted to reconstruct the maxilla by use of onlay bone grafts. They also attempted to install implants in the hip bone for subsequent transferral of the bone/implant complex to the upper jaw. Extensive problems arose with respect to implant positioning of the superstructure. After time, bone grafts in the form of horseshoe shaped onlays were attached to the alveolar bone of the deficient maxilla by the implants themselves. Attention was also paid to augment the maxilla with particulated bone (Breine & Brånemark 1988).

The onlay graft technique has been slightly modified by different groups and by the use of one-stage surgery, where implants and bone grafts are placed simultaneously. Studies have demonstrated success and survival rates of 60–80% depending on the technique used and prophylactic measures taken (Donovan *et al.* 1994; Isaksson & Alberius 1992; Jensen *et al.* 1990; Kahnberg *et al.* 1989). The major complication recorded with this method has been dehiscence of the flap with bone graft exposure and late loss of surgical implants. The need to cover the bone graft with a thick enough flap remains one of the more difficult problems. It has also been noted that a low bone-to-implant contact is achieved after four months healing although loading of implants was generally performed after six months (Nyström *et al.* 1993a).

Experimental studies have later shown the advantage in doing a two-stage procedure to allow the bone graft to be revascularized before implant insertion. Despite the relatively low success rate of onlay grafts in the total reconstruction of the jaw, these onlay grafts are indicated when treating vertical defects in the jaw or to increase the width of a thin alveolar process. An important technical surgical development has, as with orthognathic surgical methods, been the use of inlay grafts in the maxilla (Boyne *et al.* 1980; Hall *et al.* 1991; Jensen *et al.* 1992). Inlay bone grafts in the maxilla, either as local sinus lifting procedures or together with maxillary osteotomies, are used more frequently today than onlay grafts in the severely resorbed maxilla (Kahnberg *et al.* 1999; Keller 1992; Isaksson *et al.* 1993).

Sinus lifting is used mainly when there still is a residual dentition in the maxillary anterior area with insufficient bone volume beneath the sinus cavity. Sinus lifting procedures have traditionally been carried out as one-step procedures, simultaneously inserting bone graft and implants. Success and survival figures for the one-stage procedure have varied from 50% up to 90% although not all publications have provided a description of the preoperative bone volume beneath the sinus cavity. As indicated in experimental studies (Rasmusson *et al.* 1999a, b, c), a better success rate can be achieved by two-stage techniques allowing the bone graft to revascularize before implant placement. Both block graft and particulate bone as well as bone substitutes have been used in this procedure (Kent & Block 1989; Misch 1987; Moy *et al.* 1993; Kahnberg *et al.* 1989). The success and survival rates vary depending on type of graft and substitute as well as the technique used.

The interpositional bone graft used in connection with maxillary osteotomies has had a highly predictable outcome (Kahnberg *et al.* 1999; Isaksson *et al.* 1993). One-stage and two-stage techniques have been used. The one-stage technique has certain disadvantages such as implant positioning and a higher risk of implant failures (Sailer 1989). Two-stage techniques have more favorable results. An advantage with the maxillary osteotomy is that it offers the possibility to raise and lower the maxilla in order to correct sagittal discrepancies.

Increasing interest has been focused on the technique of distraction osteogenesis. It is possible to increase bone volume by slowly moving a bone segment in the desired vertical direction. In the maxilla it is especially useful when there is a local defect needing augmentation. Using this method it is possible to avoid grafting and a secondary donor site. Disadvantages include a long treatment period and instrumentation in the mouth, which is unpleasant for the patient. However, for certain cases indicated it may be a very useful method, although further studies are needed to ascertain its full potential.

## Conclusion

The reconstruction techniques of today using bone graft, orthognathic surgery or bone distraction provides the surgical specialist with a wide range of treatment options. Using these methods in an appropriate way it is possible to treat any patient with bone deficient jaws, however complicated the situation may be.

# References


Adell, R., Lekholm, U., Rockler, B. & Brånemark, P.-I. (1981) A 15-year study of osseointegrated implants in the treatment of the edentulous jaw. *Int. J. Oral Surg.* **10**:387–416.

Adell, R., Eriksson, B., Lekholm, U., Brånemark, P.-I. & Jemt, T. (1990a) A long-term follow-up study of osseointegrated implants in the fully edentulous jaws. *Int. J. Oral Maxillofac. Implants* **5**:347–359.

Adell, R., Lekholm, U., Gröndahl, K., Brånemark, P.-I., Lindström, J. & Jacobsson, M. (1990b) Reconstruction of severely resorbed edentulous maxillae using osseointegrated fixtures in immediate autogenous bone grafts. *Int. J. Oral Maxillofac. Implants* **5**:233–246.

Albrektsson, T. (1980) The healing of autologous grafts varying degrees of surgical trauma. *J. Bone Joint Surg.* **62B**:403–410.

Albrektsson, T. (1980) Repair of bone grafts. A vital microscopic and histological investigation. *Scand. J. Plast. Reconstr. Surg.* **14**:1–12.

Albrektsson, T., Brånemark, P.-I., Hansson, H.-A., Ivarsson, B. & Jönsson, U. (1982) Ultrastructural analysis of the interface zone of titanium and gold implants. *Advances in Biomat.* **4**:167–177.

Albrektsson, T., Hansson, H.-A. & Ivarsson, B. (1985) Interface analysis of titanium and zirkonium bone implants. *Biomaterials* **6**:97–101.

Albrektsson, T., Zarb, G.A., Worthington, P. & Eriksson, A.R. (1986) The long-term efficiency of currently used dental implants: A review and proposed criteria of success. *Int. J. Oral Maxillofac. Impl.* **1**:11–25.

Albrektsson, T., Eriksson, A.R., Friberg, B., Lekholm, U., Lindahl, L., Nevins, M., Oikarinen, V., Roos, J., Sennerby, L. & Åstrand, P. (1993) Histologic investigations on 33 retrieved Nobrelpharma implants. *Clin. Mat.* **122**:1–9.

Arvidson, K., Bystedt, H., Frykholm, A., von Konow, L. & Lothigius, E. (1998) Five-year prospective follow-up report of the Astra Tech Dental Implants System in the treatment of edentulous mandibles. *Clin. Oral Impl. Res.* **9**:225–234.

Boyne, P.J. & James, R.A. (1980) Grafting of the maxillary sinus floor with autogenous marrow and bone. *J. Oral Surg.* **38**:613–616.

Breine, U. & Brånemark, P.-I. Reconstuction of alveolar jaw bone. (1988) An experimental and clinical study of immediate and performed autologous bone grafts in combination with osseointegrated implants. *Scand. J. Plast. Reconstr. Surg.* **14**:23–48.

Buser, D., Schenk, R.K., Steinmann, S., Fiorellini, J.P., Fox, C.H. & Stich, H. (1991) Influence of surface characteristics on bone integration of titanium implants. A histomorphometric study in miniature. *J. Biomed. Mater. Res.* **25**:889–902.

Donovan, M.G., Dickerson, N.C., Hanson, L.J. & Gustafson, R.B. (1994) Maxillary and mandibular reconstruction using calvarial bone grafts and Brånemark implants. *J. Oral Maxillofac. Surg.* **52**:588–594.

Goldberg, V.M., Stevenson, S., Feighan, J. & Davy, D. (1995) Biology of grit-blasted titanium alloy implants. *Clin. Orthop. Rel. Res.* **319**:122–129.

Gordh, M. (1998) Survival of onlay bone grafts. A study in the adult rat. Thesis, Lund University.

Gotfredsen, K., Wennerberg, A., Johanson, C., Teil-Skovgaard, L. & Hjørting-Hansen, E. (1995) Anchorage of $TiO_2$-blasted, HA-coated, and machined implants: An experimental study with rabbit. *J. Biomed. Mater. Res.* **29**:1223–1231.

Hall, H.D. & McKenna, S.J. (1991) Bone graft of the maxillary sinus floor for Brånemark implants: A preliminary report. In: *Oral and Maxillofacial Surgery Clinics* (Eds. Worthington, P. & Breine, O.R.) Saunders: Philadelphia, pp. 869–873.

Henry, P., Laney, W., Jemt, T., Haris, D., Krogh, P., Polizzi, G., Zarb, G. & Herrmann, I. (1996) Osseointegrated implants for single-tooth replacement: A prospective 5-year multicenter study. *Int. J. Oral Maxillofac. Impl.* **11**:450–455.

Isaksson, S. & Alberius, P. (1992) Maxillary alveolar ridge augmentation with onlay bone-grafts and immediate endosseous implants. *J. Craniomaxillofac. Surg.* **20**:2–7.

Isaksson, S., Ekfeldt, A., Alberius, P. & Blomqvist, J.E. (1993) Early results from reconstruction of severely atrophic (class VI) maxillas by immediate endosseous implants in conjunction with bone grafting and Le Fort I osteotomy. *J. Oral Maxillofac. Surg.* **22**:144–148.

Jensen, O.T. & Sennerby, L. (1998) Histologic analysis of clinically retrieved titanium microimplants placed in conjunction with maxillary sinus floor augmentation. *Int. J. Oral Maxillofac. Impl.* **13**:513–521.

Jensen, J., Krantz Simonsen, E. & Sindet-Pedersen, S. (1990) Reconstruction of the severely resorbed maxilla with bone grafting and osseointegrated implants: A preliminary report. *J. Oral Maxillofac. Surg.* **48**:27–32.

Jensen, O.T., Perkins, S. & Van de Water, F.W. (1992) Nasal fossa and maxillary sinus grafting of implants from a palatal approach: Report of a case. *J. Oral Maxillofac. Surg.* **50**:415–418.

Kahnberg, K.-E., Nystrom, E. & Bartholdsson, L. (1989) Combined use of bone grafts and Brånemark fixtures in the treatment of severely resorbed maxillae. *Int. J. Maxillofac. Implants* **4**:297–304.

Kahnberg, K.-E., Nilsson, P. & Rasmusson, L. (1999) Le Fort I Osteotomy with Interpositional Bone Grafts and Implants for Rehabilitation of the Severely Resorbed Maxilla: A 2-Stage Procedure. *Int. J. Oral Maxillofac. Implants* **14**:571–578.

Keller, E.E. (1992) The maxillary interpositional composite graft (LeFort I Osteotomy with interpositional autogenous iliac bone graft and titanium endosseous implants). In: *Advanced Osseointegration Surgery: Applications in the Maxillofacial Region.* (Eds. Worthington, P. & Brånemark, P.I.) Quintessence, Chicago, Illinois, p. 162.

Kent, J.N. & Block, M.S. (1989) Simultaneous maxillary sinus floor bone grafting and placement of hydoxyapatite-coated implants. *J. Oral Maxillofac. Surg.* **47**:238–242.

Lekholm, U., van Steenberghe, D., Herrmann, I., Bolender, C., Folmer, T., Gunne, J., Henry, P., Higuchi, K., Laney, W.R. & Lindén, U. (1994) Osseointegrated implants in the treatment of partially edentulous jaws. A prospective 5-year multicenter study. *Int. J. Oral Maxillofac. Implants* **9**:627–635.

Lew, D., Marino, A.A., Startzell, J.M. & Keller, J.C. (1994) A comparative study of osseointegration of titanium implants in corticocancellous block and corticocancellous chip grafts in canine ileum. *J. Oral Maxillofac. Surg.* **52**:952–958.

Linder, L., Obrant, K. & Boivin, G. (1989) Osseointegration of metallic implants. II. Transmission electron microscopy in the rabbit. *Acta Orthop. Scand.* **60**:35–139.

Makkonen, T.A., Holmberg, S., Niemi, L., Olsson, C., Tammisalo, T. & Peltola, J.A. (1997) 5-year prospective clinical study of Astra Tech dental implants supporting fixed bridges or overdentures in the edentulous mandible. *Clin. Oral Impl. Res.* **8**:469–475.

Meredith, N., Cawley, P. & Alleyne, D. (1996a) Quantitative determination of the stability of the implant/tissue interface using Resonance Frequency Analysis. *Clin. Oral Impl. Res.* **7**:261–267.

Meredith, N., Rasmusson, L., Sennerby, L. & Alleyne, D. (1996b) Mapping implant stability by resonance frequency analysis. *Med. Sci. Res.* **24**:191–193.

Misch, C.E. (1987) Maxillary sinus augmentation for endosteal implants: Organized alternative treatment plans. *Int. J. Oral Implantology* **4**:49–58.

Moy, P.K., Lundgren, S. & Holmes, RE. (1993) Maxillary sinus augmentation: histomorphometric analysis of graft materials for maxillary sinus floor augmentation. *J. Oral Maxillofac. Surg.* **51**:857–862.

Nanci, A., McCarthy, G.F., Zalzal, S., Clokie, C.M.L., Warshawsky, H. & McKee, M.D. (1994) Tissue response to titanium implants in the rat tibia: ultrastructural, immunocytochemical and lectin-cytochemical characterization of the bone-titanium interface. *Cells and Materials* **4**:1–30.

Neukam, F.W., Scheller, H. & Günay, H. (1989) Experimentelle und klinische Untersuchungen zur Auflagerungsosteoplastik in Kombination mit enossalen Implantaten. *Z. Zahnärztl. Implantol.* **5**:235–241.

Nyström, E., Kahnberg, K.-E. & Gunne, J. (1993) Bone grafts and Brånemark implants in the treatment of the severely resorbed maxilla: A 2-year longitudinal study. *Int. J. Oral Maxillofac. Implants* **8**:45–53.

Nyström, E., Kahnberg, K.-E. & Albrektsson, T. (1993) Treatment of the Severely Resorbed Maxillae With Bone Graft and Titanium Implants: Histologic Review of Autopsy Specimens. *Int. J. Oral Maxillofac. Implants* **8**:167–172.

O'Sullivan, D., Sennerby, L. & Meredith, N. (2000) Measurements comparing the initial stability of five designs of dental implants: a human cadaver study. *Clin. Implant Dent. Relat. Res.* **2**:85–92.

Pinholt, E.M., Haanaes, H.R., Roervik, M., Donath, K. & Bang, G. (1992) Alveolar ridge augmentation by osteoinductive materials in goats. *Scand. J. Dent. Res.* **100**:361–365.

Piatelli, A., Degidi, M., Marchetti, C. & Scarano, A. (1997) Histologic analysis of the interface of a titanium implant retrieved from a nonvascularized mandibular block graft after a 10-month loading period. *Int. J. Oral Maxillofac. Impl.* **12**:840–843.

Rasmusson, L., Meredith, N., Kahnberg, K.-E. & Sennerby, L. (1998) Stability assessments and histology of titanium implants placed simultaneously with autogenous onaly bone in the rabbit tibia. *Int. J. Oral Maxillofac. Surg.* **27**:229–235.

Rasmusson, L., Meredith, N., Kahnberg, K.-E. & Sennerby, L. (1999) Effects of barrier membranes on bone resorption and implant stability in onlay bone grafts. An experimental study. *Clin. Oral Impl. Res.* **10**:267–277.

Rasmusson, L., Stegersjö, G., Kahnberg, K.-E. & Sennerby, L. (1999) Implant Stability Measurements Using Resonance Frequency Analysis in the Grafted Maxilla: A Cross-Sectional Pilot Study. *Clin. Impl. Dent. Relat. Res.* **1**:70–74.

Rasmusson, L., Meredith, N., Cho, I.H. & Sennerby, L. (1999) The influence of simultaneous vs delayed placement on the stability of titanium implants in onlay bone grafts. A histologic and biomechanic study in the rabbit. *Int. J. Oral Maxillofac. Surg.* **28**:224–231.

Rosen, P., Summers, R., Mellado, J.R., Salkin, L.M., Shanaman, R.H., Marks, H. M. & Fugazotto, P.A. (1999) The bone-added osteotome sinus floor elevation technique: multicenter retrospective report of consecutively treated patients. *Int. J. Oral Maxillofac. Surg.* **14:** 853–858.

Sailer, H.F. (1989) A new method of inserting endosseous implants in totally atrophic maxillae. *J. Craniomaxillofac. Surg.* **17**:299–305.

Sennerby, L., Thomsen, P. & Ericson, L.E. (1992) A biomechanical and morphometric comparison of titanium implants inserted in rabbit cortical and cancellous bone in rabbits. *Int. J. Oral Maxillofac. Implants* **7**:62–71.

Sennerby, L., Thomsen, P. & Ericson, L.E. (1993) Early response to titanium implants inserted in rabbit in cortical bone. Part I: Light microscopic observations. *J. Mater. Sci. Mater. Med.* **4**:240–250.

Shirota, T., Ohno, K., Michi, K.-I. & Tachikawa, T. (1991) An experimental study of healing around hydroxyapatite implants installed with autogenous iliac bone grafts for jaw reconstruction. *J. Oral Maxillofac. Surg.* **49**:1310–1315.

Smith, J.D. & Abrahamson, M. (1974) Membranous vs enchondral bone autografts. *Arch Otolaryngol.* **99**:203–207.

Wennerberg, A. (1996) *On surface roughness and implant incorporation.* Thesis, Göteborg University, Göteborg, Sweden.

Zellin, G. (1988) Growth factors and bone regeneration. Implications of barrier membranes. *Swed. Dent. J.* **Suppl 129**, pp. 7–65.

# Further Reading


Åhrén, S. & Kahnberg, K.-E. (2001) The Adaptation of Implant-Supported Superstructures to the Alveolar Crest: A Follow-Up of 49 Cases. *Implant Dent.* **10**:172–177.

Albrektsson, T. (1981) A microangiographic representation of the microvascular system in bone tissue. A vital microscopic evaluation in the rabbit. *Clin. Orthop. Rel. Res.* **159**:268–275.

Albrektsson, T. (1981) Ischaemia and bone graft. *Scand. J. Plast. Reconstr. Surg.* **19** (suppl 16):21–24.

Albrektsson, T. & Lindner, L. (1981) A method of short and long term in vivo study of the bone implant interface. *Clin. Orthop. Rel. Res.* **159**:251–255.

Albrektsson, T. & Lindner, L. (1981) Intravital, long-term followup of autologous experimental bone grafts. *Archiv. Orthop. Traumat. Surg.* **98**:189–193.

Bell, C.S., Thrash, W.J. & Zysset, H.K. (1986) Incidence of maxillary sinusitis following LeFort I Osteotomy. *J. Oral Maxillofac. Surg.* **44**:100–103.

Burchardt, H. & Enneking, W.F. (1978) Transplantation of bone. *Surg. Clin. North Am.* **58**:403–427.

Burchardt, H. (1983) Biology of cortical bone graft incorporation. In: *Osteochondral Allografts – Biology, Banking and Clinical Applications.* (Eds. Friedlander, H. & Mankin, H.) Little Brown & Co. Boston, MA, USA, pp. 51–57.

Cawood, J.I. & Howell, RA. (1990) Reconstructive preprosthetic surgery. Anatomical considerations. *Int. J. Oral Maxillofac. Surg.* **20**:75–82.

Cawood, J.I., Stoelinga, P.J.W. & Brouns, J.J.A. (1994) Reconstruction of a severely resorbed (Class VI) maxilla: a two-step procedure. *Int. J. Oral Maxillofac. Surg.* **23**:219–225.

DeLacure, M.D. Physiology of bone healing and bone grafts. (1994) *Otolaryngol. Clin. North Am.* **27**:859–874.

Farrell, C.D., Kent, J.N. & Guerra, LR. (1976) One-stage interpositional bone grafting and vestibuloplasty of the atrophic maxilla. *J. Oral Surg.* **34**:901–906.

Gilbert, A. (1979) Vascularized transfer of the fibular shaft. *Int. J. Microsurg.* **1**:100–102.

Gunne, J., Nyström, E. & Kahnberg, K.-E. (1995) Bone Grafts and Implants in the Treatment of the Severely Resorbed Maxillae: A 3-Year Follow-up of the Prosthetic Restoration. *Int. J. Prosthodont.* **8**:38–45.

Hardesty, R.A. & Marsh, J.L. (1990) Craniofacial onlay bone grafting: A prospective evaluation of graft morphology, orientation, and embryonic origin. *Plast. Reconstr. Surg.* **85**:5–14.

Heiple, K.G., Chase, S.W. & Hernon, C.H. (1963) A comparative study of the healing process following different types of bone transplantation. *J. Bone Joint Surg.* **45A**:1593–1616.

Hollinger, J.O. (1993) Factors for osseous repair and delivery: Part I. *J. Craniofac. Surg.* **4**:102–108.

Hollinger, J.O. (1993) Strategies for regenerating bone of the craniofacial complex. *Bone* **14**:575–580.

Holmes, R.E. & Hagler, H.K. (1988) Porous hydroxylapatite as a bone graft substitute in maxillary augmentation. A histometric study. *J. Craniomaxillofac. Surg.* **16**:199–205.

Jensen, J., Sindet-Pedersen, S. & Oliver, A.J. (1994) Varying treatment strategies for reconstruction of maxillary atrophy with implants. Results in 98 patients. *J. Oral Maxillofac. Surg.* **52**:210–216.

Kahnberg, K.-E., Rasmusson, L. & Mohammadi, S. (1998) An experimental rabbit model for studying the healing of onlay bone grafts. *Swed. Dent. J.* **22**:15–21.

Kahnberg, K.-E., Ekestubbe, A., Gröndahl, K., Nilsson, P. & Hirsch, J.-M. (2001) Sinus lifting procedure. I. One-stage surgery with bone transplant and implants. *Clin. Oral Impl. Res.* **12**:479–487.

Keller, E.E., Van Roeckel, N.B., Desjardins, R.P. & Tolman, D.E. (1987) Prosthetic reconstruction of the severely resorbed maxilla with iliac grafting and tissue-integrated prostheses. *Int. J. Oral Maxillofac. Implants* **2**:155–165.

Keller, E.E. & Sather, A.H. (1990) Quadrangular LeFort I osteotomy: Surgical technique and review of 54 patients. *J. Oral Maxillofac. Surg.* **48**:2–11.

Keller, E.E. & Tolman, D.E. (1991) Mandibular ridge augmentation with simultaneous onlay iliac bone graft and endosseous implants: A preliminary report. *Int. J. Maxillofac. Implants* **7**:176–184.

Keller, E.E. & Triplet, W.W. (1987) Iliac bone grafting: Review of 160 consecutive cases. *J. Oral Maxillofac. Surg.* **45**:11–14.

Keller, E.E., Tolman, D.E. & Brånemark, P.I. (1992) Surgical reconstruction of advanced maxillary resorption with composite grafts (autogenous iliac bone and endosseous titanium implants). In: *Advanced Osseointegration Surgery: Applications in the Maxillofacial Region.* (Eds. Worthington, P. & Brånemark, P.I.) Quintessence, Chicago, Illinois, pp. 146–161.

Keller, E.E., Eckert, S.E. & Tolman, D.E. (1994) Maxillary antral and nasal one-stage inlay composite bone graft. Preliminary report on 30 recipient sites. *J. Oral Maxillofac. Surg.* **52**:438–448.

La Trenta, G.S., McCarthy, J.G., Breitbart, A.S., May, M. & Sissons, H.A. (1989) The role of rigid fixation in bone-graft augmentation of the craniofacial skeleton. *Plast. Reconstr. Surg.* **84**:578–588.

Lew, D., Hinkle, R.M., Unhold, G.P. *et al.* (1991) Reconstruction of the severely atrophic edentulous mandible by means of autogenous bone grafts and simultaneous placement of osseointegrated implants. *J. Oral Maxillofac. Surg.* **49**:228–233.

Lin, K.Y., Bartlett, S.P., Yaremchuk, M.J., Fallon, M., Grossmanet, R.F. & Whitaker, L.A. (1990) The effect of rigid fixation on the survival of onlay bone grafts: An experimental study. *Plast. Reconstr. Surg.* **86**:449–456.

Liström, R.D. & Symington, J.M. (1988) Osseointegrated dental implants in conjunction with bone grafts. *Int. J. Oral Maxillofac. Surg.* **47**:116–118.

Loukota, R.A., Isaksson, S.G., Linnér, E.L.J. & Blomqvist, J.E. (1992) A technique for inserting endosseous implants in the atrophic maxilla in a single stage procedure. *Br. J. Oral Maxillofac. Surg.* **30**:46–49.

Lozada, J.L., Emanuelli, S., James, R.A., Boskovic, M. & Lindsted, K. (1993) Implants placed in subanthral grafted sites. *J. Calif. Dent. Assoc.* **21**:31–35.

Lozano, A.J., Cestero, H.J. & Salyer, K.E. (1976) The early revascularisation of onlay bone grafts. *Plast. Reconstr. Surg.* **58**:302–305.

Lyberg, T. & Olstad, O.A. (1991) The vascularized fibular flap for mandibular reconstruction. *J. Craniomaxillofac. Surg.* **19**:113–118.

Marx, R.E. & Morales, M.J. (1988) Morbidity from bone harvested in major jaw reconstruction. A randomized trial comparing the lateral anterior and posterior approaches to the ilium. *J. Oral Maxillofac. Surg.* **48**:196–203.

Mohammadi, S., Rasmusson, L., Göransson, L., Sennerby, L., Thomsen, P. & Kahnberg, K.-E. (2000) Healing of titanium implants in onlay bone grafts: an experimental rabbit model. *J. Mater. Sci. Mater. Med.* **11**:83–89.

Nyström, E., Legrell, P.E., Forssell, Å. & Kahnberg, K.-E. (1995) Combined use of bone grafts and implants in the severely resorbed maxilla. Postoperative evaluation by computed tomography. *Int. J. Oral Maxillofac. Surg.* **24**:20–25.

Nyström, E., Ahlqvist, J., Kahnberg, K.-E. & Rosenquist, J.B. (1996) Autogenous onlay bone grafts fixed with screw implants for the treatment of severely resorbed maxillae. Radiographic evaluation of preoperative bone dimensions, postoperative bone loss, and changes in soft-tissue profile. *Int. J. Oral Maxillofac. Surg.* **25**:351–359.

Nyström, E., Ahlqvist, J., Legrell, P.E. & Kahnberg, K.-E. (2002) Bone graft remodelling and implant success rate in the treatment of the severely resorbed maxilla: a 5-year longitudinal study. *Int. J. Oral Maxillofac. Surg.* **31**:158–164.

Nyström, E., Ahlqvist, J. & Kahnberg, K.-E. (in publication) 10-year Follow-up of Onlay Bone Grafts and Implants in Severely Resorbed Maxillae.

Quiney, R.E., Brimble, E. & Hodge, M. (1990) Maxillary sinusitis from dental osseointegrated implants. *J. Laryngol. Otol.* **104**:333–334.

Raghoebar, G.M., Brouwer, T.J., Reintsema, H. & Van Oort, R.P. (1993) Augmentation of the maxillary sinus floor with autogenous bone for the placement of endosseous implants. *J. Oral Maxillofac. Surg.* **51**:1198–1203.

Rasmusson, L., Kahnberg, K.-E. & Tan, A. (2001) Effect of implant design and surface on bone regeneration and implant stability: an experimental study in the dog mandible. *Clin. Impl. Dent. Relat. Res.* **3**:2–8.

Riediger, D. (1988) Restoration of masticatory function by microsurgically revascularized iliac crest bone grafts using endosseous implants. *Plast. Reconstr. Surg.* **81**:861–876.

Salata, L.Z., Rasmusson, L. & Kahnberg, K.-E. (2002) Effects of a mechanical barrier on the integration of cortical onlay bone grafts placed simultaneously with endosseous implant. *Clin. Impl. Dent. Relat. Res.* **4**:60–68.

Serra, J.M., Paloma, V., Mesa, F. & Ballesteros, A. (1991) The vascularized fibula graft in mandibular reconstruction. *J. Oral Maxillofac. Surg.* **49**:244–250.

Sindet-Pedersen, S. & Enemark, H. (1990) Reconstruction of alveolar clefts with mandibular or iliac crest bone grafts. A comparative study. *J. Oral Maxillofac. Surg.* **48**:554–558.

Small, S.A., Zinner, I.D., Panno, F.V., Shapiro, H.J. & Stein, J.I. (1993) Augmenting the maxillary sinus for implants: Report of 27 patients. *Int. J. Oral Maxillofac. Implants* **8**:523–528.

Smiler, D.G. & Holmes, R.E. (1987) Sinus lift procedure using porous hydroxyapatite: A preliminary clinical report. *J. Oral Implantol.* **13**:239–253.

Smiler, D.G., Johnson, P.W., Loyada, J.L., Misch, C., Rosenlicht, J.L., Tatum, O.H. Jr & Wagner, J.R. (1992) Sinus lift grafts and endosseous implants. Treatment of the atrophic posterior maxilla. *Dent. Clin. North Am.* **36**:151–186.

Stevenson, S., Emery, S.E. & Goldberg, V.M. (1996) Factors affecting bone graft incorporation. *Clin. Orthop. Rel. Res.* **324**:66–74.

Tatum, H. Jr (1986) Maxillary and sinus implant reconstruction. *Dent. Clin. North Am.* **30**:207–229.

Tidwell, J.K., Blijdorp, P.A., Stoelinga, W. *et al.* (1992) Composite grafting of the maxillary sinus for placement of endosteal implants. A preliminary report of 48 patients. *Int. J. Oral Maxillofac. Surg.* **21**:204–209.

Ueda, M. & Kaneda, T. (1992) Maxillary sinusitis caused by dental implants. Report of two cases. *J. Oral Maxillofac. Surg.* **50**:285–287.

Wood, R.M. & Moore, D.L. (1988) Grafting of the maxillary sinus with intraorally harvested autogenous bone prior to implant placement. *Int. J. Oral Maxillofac. Implants* **3**:209–213.

Yaszemski, M.J., Payne, R.G., Hayes, W.C., Langer, R. & Mikos, A.G. (1996) Evolution of bone transplantation: Molecular, cellular and tissue strategies to engineer human bone. *Biomaterials* **17**:175–185.

# Index

Page numbers in *italics* refer to figures.


abdominal cavity perforations, 69
abutment connection
  major onlay grafts, 23
  minor onlay grafts, 19
  sinus lift grafts, 37, *37*
  *see also* closure techniques *or* healing
acrylic stents, *25*
allografts
  defined, 1
alveolar bone impaction techniques, 47, *47*
alveolar nerve, 69
  avoidance techniques, 14, 15–16, *16*
alveolar process reconstruction
  alveolar impaction into maxillary sinus, 47, *47*
  distraction osteogenesis, 63, *63–6*, 66–7
  segmental osteotomies, 57, *57–9*, 59–60, *60–61*
  split crest techniques, 20, *27–9*
alveolar process grafts, 69
alveolar process resorption, 33, *57*, *63*
angiogenesis, 2–3
antibiotics, 48
artificial bone, 1, 18, 73, *73*
  use with particulated bone, 33, 73
'autografts'
  defined, 1
  indications, 1
  sources, 1–2

bicortical onlay grafts, 8
  complications, 69
  *see also* cortico-cancellous grafts
Bio-Oss®, 18, 73, *73*
bleeding
  mandibular (mental) bone graft complications, 69
BMPs *see* bone morphogenetic proteins (BMPs)
bone collecting devices, 18, *18*, 33–4
bone mill (particulation), *17*
bone morphogenetic proteins (BMPs), 3
bone substitutes *see* artificial bone
bone-to-implant contact studies, 8–9, 75
BoneTrap™, 18, *18*, 33–4
Brånemark implants
  contact studies, 8
bridge construction, *43*, *45*, *54*, *56*, *65*
buccal
  crest widening procedures, 29, *27–9*
  onlays, 21–2, *22*, 24
    and chin grafts, 14, *22*
    indications for use, 24, 75
  ridge damage
    and major block grafts, 24

calvarial bone grafts, 34
  complications, 69
cancellous grafts
  in-growth rates for titanium implants, 7–9
  one-stage graft with multiple implants, 37, *38*
  revascularization rates, 3
ceramics, 1
chin grafts, 2, 14–15, *15*, *22*
  complications, 14
  indications for use, 14
  surgical techniques, 14–15, *15*, *22*
choralline substances, 18, 73, *73*

closure techniques
  major block grafts, 23
  minor block grafts, 21–2
  minor grafts with particulated bone, 19
  sinus lift grafts, *39*, *40*, *46*
  *see also* fixation methods *or* suturing techniques
clotting cascade, 2–3
complications
  abdominal cavity perforations, 69
  from grafting sites
    calvarial grafts, 69
    chin grafts, 14
    iliac crest grafts, 12, 69
    mandibular angle grafts, 16, 69
    mandibular mental grafts, 69
    tibial bone grafts, 13, 69
  from inlay grafts, 33, 70–71, *71*
    alveolar impaction, 47
    maxillary sinus cavity infections, 33
    oro-antral fistula formations, 71, *71*
  from onlay grafting, 21–2, 69–70, *70*
    flap dehiscence, 75
cortical grafts
  implant in-growth rates, 7–9
  maxillary osteotomies, 48
  minor block grafts, 21–2
  revascularization rates, 3
  segmental osteotomies, *57–8*, 59–60
  strength, 3
cortico-cancellous grafts
  block grafts vs particulated grafts, 8
  and graft stability, 8
  one-stage graft with multiple implants, 37, *38*
crest fractures, 69

demineralization, *28*
denture trauma, *70*
  and alveolar process resorption, 33, 47
distraction devices, *64*, 66, *67*
distraction osteogenesis, 63–7, 76
  disadvantages, 76
  indications for use, 63, 67, 76
  surgical techniques, *63–6*, 66–7, *67*

fibrous dysplasia, *60*
fibula bone, 1–2
fistula formations, 71, *71*
fixation methods
  in distraction osteogenesis procedures, *64*, 66
  in major block grafts, 23, *25*
  in maxillary osteotomies, 48, *49–50*
  and micromobility, 71
  in minor block grafts, *21*, *22*
  in minor particulated bone grafts, 19
  in nasal inlay grafts, 31, *32*
  sinus lift procedures, 33, *34*, 39, *40*, *44*, *46*, 70–71
  stability of implants, 8–9, 21–2, 23, 34–5
  use of bone substitute packing, 18, 73, *73*
  use of wire and plate screws, 39, *40–41*
  *see also* closure techniques
fracture healing, 2

gene technology, 3
graft bed preparation
  major block implants, 23
  minor block grafts, 21
graft incorporation
  principles of healing, 2–3
  remodeling response times (titanium implants), 5
grafting materials
  background history, 1
  complications, 12–14, 16, 69
  and particulated bone, 17, 19, *20–21*, 21, *22*, 33, *36*
  sites for harvesting, 1–2
  substitute bone materials, 1, 18, 73, *73*
grafting (donor) procedures, 11–17
  alveolar process grafts, 69
  chin grafts, 2, 14–15, *15*, *22*
  iliac crest grafts, 11–12, *12–13*

mandibular angle grafts, 2, 15–16, *16*, 24, 69
mandibular mental grafts, 69
maxillary tuberosity grafts, 17, 69
tibial bone grafts, 1–2, 13, *13*, 69
growth factors, new developments, 3

healing
general principles, 2–3, 5
and prosthetic loading, 23, 35, 39, *54, 56*, 70
soft tissues, *26*
stimulation techniques, 21, 23
in procedures
distraction osteogenesis, *64*, 66
maxillary osteotomies, 48, *50*, *51*
multiple implants with one-stage sinus lift, 37
nasal inlay grafts, 31
single implants with local sinus lift, 35
two-stage sinus lift and implant installation, 39, *41*, *43*, *45*
wound dehiscence, 71, 75
hematoma formation, 2, 5
hernia formation, 69
histomorphometry
defined, 7
removal torque test, 7
historical perspectives, 1
hydroxyapatite, 1, 18, 73

iliac crest grafts, 11–12, *12–13*, *14*, *25*
bone-to-implant contact studies, 8–9
calcified matrix retention, 8
complications, 12, 69
indications for use, 11
medial vs lateral sites, 11–12
postoperative morbidity, 12
surgical technique, 11–12, *12–13*
Implant Stability Quotient (ISQ) units, *6*
implants
bone formation responses, 5–6
comparison of materials, *6*, *7*
installation, 8–9, 21–2, 23–4
following distraction osteogenesis, *64–5*, 67
following major block grafts, 23, *25–7*
following maxillary osteotomy, 48, *52–4*
following minor block grafts, 21–2
following sinus lift with grafting, 39, *41–5*
with local sinus lift, 34–5, *35–7*
with segmental osteotomies, *59*, *61*
with sinus lift and block grafting, 37, *38*
morphological studies, 6
postoperative complications, 69–71, 75
revascularization considerations, 2–3, 75
stability comparisons (grafted/non-grafted bone), 8–9, *9*
and surface roughness, 6
surgical guide pins, *41*, *45*
use of bone substitute packing, 73, *73*
*see also* titanium implants
inferior alveolar nerve, 69
avoidance techniques, 14, 15–16, *16*
inflammatory response, 2–3
inlay grafts
complications, 70–71, *71*, 76
indications for use, 76
maxilla osteotomy with interpositional bone graft, 47–8, *48*, *49–56*
maxillary sinus alveolar impaction, 47, *47*
nasal inlay grafting, 31, *32*
sinus lift procedures, 33–46
one-stage multiple implants, 37, *38–9*
one-stage single implants, 34–5, *35–7*
two-stage processes, 39, *40–46*
interpositional bone graft procedures, 47–8, *48*, *49–56*, 76
complications 47, *47*
healing rates, 48, *50*, *51*

Lindemann bur, 13, 15
loading *see* prosthetic loading

major onlay block grafts, 23–9
  complications, 21–2, 69–70, *70*, 75
  and implants, 24, *25–7*
  indications for use, 23, 75
  prosthetic loading, 75
  success rates, 23, 75
mandibular angle grafts, 2, 15–16
  complications, 16, 69
  indications for use, 15, 24
  surgical technique, 15–16, *16*
mandibular mental grafts
  complications, 69
maxillary osteotomies, 76
  healing rates, 48, *50*, *51*
  interpositional bone graft procedures, 47–8, *48*, *49–56*
maxillary sinus grafting *see* sinus lift procedures
maxillary sinus infections, 33
maxillary tuberosity grafts, 17
  complications, 69
  indications for use, 17
micromobility, 71
minor onlay block grafts, 21–2, *22*
  indications for use, 21
  surgical techniques, 21–2, *22*
mucosa integrity, 33

nasal inlay grafts, 31, *32*
  indications for use, 31
  surgical technique, *32*
nasal mucosa perforations, 70
neuralgic pain
  chin graft harvesting, 14
  mandibular bone grafts, 69

one-stage grafting techniques, 75
  complications, 75
  with multiple implants, 37, *38–9*
  with single implants, 34–5, *35–7*
onlay grafting, 19–29, 75–6
  background history, 75–6
  complications, 69–70, *70*, 75
  healing times, 19, *20–21*, 21–2, 23
  indications for use, 19, 75
  major grafts in block form, 23–9
  minor grafts in block form, 21–2, *22*
  minor grafts with particulated bone, 19, *20–21*
  prosthetic loading, 75
  surgical techniques, 19, *20*
oro-antral fistula formations, 71, *71*
osteogenic response, 2
osteosutures
  maxillary osteotomies, 48, *49–50*
  sinus lift procedures, 39, *40–41*, *44*, *46*
osteotomes, 47, *47*
osteotomy techniques
  for maxilla atrophy, 47–8, *48*, *49–51*
  segmental procedures for bone augmentation, 57, *57–9*, 59–60, *60–61*
  'window' procedures, 35, *35*, 37, *38*

packing techniques, *20*, *22*
  *see also* particulated bone
pain, 69
  *see also* inferior alveolar nerve
palatal mucosa (upper jaw)
  distraction vs segmentation, 67
particulated bone
  and artificial bone mix ratios, 33
  as onlay graft material, 19, *20–21*
  as packing, 21, *22*, *36*
  in sinus lift procedures, 33, *36*
  techniques and equipment (bone mill), *17*
periosteum integrity, 66
plastics, 1
postoperative complications *see* complications
prosthetic loading, 23
  complications, 70
  timescales, *54*, *56*
    onlay bone grafts, 75

single implants with local sinus lift, 35
two-stage sinus lift procedures, 39
proteins, bone morphogenetic proteins (BMPs), 3
pseudarthroses, 70

recombinant techniques, 3
remodelling
morphological studies, 6
and surface roughness, 6
timescales, 5
*see also* healing
removal torque test, 7
implant integration studies, 8–9, *9*
research
bone-to-implant contact studies, 8–9, 75
implant integration studies, 8–9
titanium implant morphological studies, 6
resonance frequency analysis (RFA), *6*, 7
implant integration studies, 8–9
resorption, upper jaw, *49*, *51*
revascularization considerations
cancellous grafts, 3
cortical grafts, 3
and implant stability, 2–3, 75–6
rib grafts, 1–2

Safe Scraper, 18
Scanora tomography, *55*
segmental osteotomies, 57–61
indications for use, 57
surgical techniques, *58–9*, 59–60, *61*
single implants with local sinus lift, 34–5, *35–7*
sinus lift procedures, 33–46, 76
choice of donor site, 11, 13, 14, 33–4
complications, 70–71, *71*
drainage problems, 33
indications for use, 76
infection risk, 33
and nasal inlay grafts, 31
one-stage multiple implants, 37, *38–9*, 75
one-stage single implants, 34–5, *35–7*
two-stage processes, 39, *40–46*, 75–6
use of particulated bone, 33
sinus membrane integrity, 33, 70–71
sinusitis, 70, *71*
sources for bones grafts, 1–2
*see also* grafting (donor) procedures
split crest techniques
alveolar process reconstruction, 29, *27–9*
stabilization *see* fixation methods
surface roughness, 6
surgical guide pins, *41*, *45*
suturing techniques
following distraction osteogenesis, *64*
one-stage sinus lift with multiple implants, *39*
onlay grafts, 19
two-stage sinus lift with multiple implants, *40*, *46*
*see also* closure techniques

terminology, 1
tibial bone grafts, 1–2, 13
complications, 13, 69
indications for use, 13
surgical technique, 13, *13*
tissue regeneration, new developments, 3
titanium implants
bone formation responses, 5–6
morphological studies, 6
osteointegration in block v. particulated grafts, 8
removal torque test studies, 7–9
resonance frequency analysis (RFA), 7–9
simultaneous vs delayed placements, 8–9
surface roughness, 6
*see also* implants

trephination, 1
trephine drill techniques
  chin grafts, *15*
  *see also* grafting (donor) procedures
two-stage sinus lift grafts, 39, *40–46*, 75–6
  indications for use, 39, 75
  surgical technique, 39, *40–46*

vascularization, 2
  of cancellous grafts, 3
  of cortical grafts, 3
  and implant stability, 75–6
von Walter, Dr Philip, 1

window technique, 37, *38*
  *see also* grafting (donor) procedures
wound dehiscence, *71*, 75
woven bone, formation, 5–6

xenografts, 1